SICK SKIN

SKINCARE MADE SIMPLE

YUVAL BIBI, MD, PHD

BOARD-CERTIFIED DERMATOLOGIST

Disclaimer: Neither the publisher nor the author engages in rendering professional, health, medical advice, or services to the individual reader. This book is designed to provide general information for our readers. This book is not meant to be used, nor should it be used, to diagnose or treat any medical condition. The author does not intend for the ideas, procedures, and suggestions contained in this book to be a substitute for consulting with your physician. All matters regarding your health require medical supervision. Neither the author nor the publisher shall be liable or responsible for any loss or damage allegedly arising from any information or suggestion in this book.

Prominence Publishing

www.prominencepublishing.com

The author can be reached as follows: https://drbibiorganics.com

Cover design by Prominence Publishing, Inc.

Sick Skin/Yuval Bibi. -- 1st ed.

ISBN: 978-1-990830-29-7

Dedicated with love to my parents,

Dr. Haim Bibi, a man of medicine, tenacity, and infinite good will,
and Nili Bibi, a woman of creativity, generosity, and grit.

ACKNOWLEDGMENTS

The journey of writing this book spanned over five years, but its foundations were built upon years of training, studying, and working with numerous patients, mentors, and colleagues. Countless discussions and insights, though not directly included in the book, significantly influenced my understanding of medicine, dermatology, skincare, and beyond.

I am indebted to Dr. Elliot J. Androphy, a distinguished dermatologist, brilliant scientist, and critical thinker, who served as my post-doctoral mentor and a true friend during my early years in the United States. Without his unwavering support and encouragement, my path in dermatology would not have been possible.

The late Dr. Amal K. Kurban, an extraordinary dermatologist who pushed everyone to excel, a true Renaissance man, and a formidable thinker, blessed me with his mentorship and enduring friendship. Many of the ideas and critiques explored in this book took shape during our animated discussions about academia, dermatology, medicine, and the human condition in his Boston University office.

Dr. Lynne J. Goldberg, a sharp and insightful clinician, as well as a generous teacher and colleague, deserves my gratitude. It was through her passion for scalp dermatology that my own interest and love for the field ignited.

Dr. Lynette J. Margesson, whom I had the privilege of meeting during my residency training in Boston, is a brilliant dermatologist. Her expertise in managing vulvovaginal disorders inspired me to specialize in genital dermatology, offering solutions and helping alleviate the suffering of countless patients.

Dr. Lisa Benest, an exceptional dermatologist, shrewd businesswoman, and dear friend, generously welcomed me to her practice when I relocated to Los Angeles. Dr. Benest's open-mindedness in tailoring treatments for each patient, her exploration of alternative healing approaches, and her healthy skepticism of institutional orthodoxy significantly influenced the points I present in this book.

During the writing process, it was imperative to discuss certain ideas with the trailblazers who paved the way.

Dr. Michael F. Holick, a medical and scientific authority, challenged the mainstream narrative through his views on sun exposure and human health. His independent thinking, common sense, meticulous analysis of research, and courage to ask difficult questions led to his perspectives being labeled "contrarian." Dr. Holick's insights on human behavior, sun exposure, and vitamin D are truly cutting-edge.

Dr. Han van der Rhee, a Dutch dermatologist, graciously engaged in discussions about crucial points raised in this book. His wisdom and comprehensive understanding of sun exposure and human health are invaluable.

Dr. Ian A. Myles, an exceptional scientist and physician, whose groundbreaking discoveries are revolutionizing our understanding of microbiology and the intricate relationship between human biology and the microbiome. Dr. Myles provided valuable contributions from his insightful perspective on the microbiome, institutions, and beyond.

Suzanne Doyle-Ingram of Prominence Publishing, my amazing publisher, worked tirelessly to bring "Sick Skin" to fruition. She took great care in shaping and preserving the essence and value of this book, while guiding me throughout the process.

I am eternally grateful to my patients. Throughout my career, I have had the privilege of actively participating in the lives of tens of thousands of patients.

I thank them for entrusting me with their care and for generously sharing their feedback and insights over the years.

Lastly, I express my gratitude to God for blessing my life with these wonderful individuals, providing me with the strength to write this book, and granting me the courage to share it with the world.

Table of Contents

Preface

Learn to speak *Skinese*, the language of your skin. Reclaim agency over your skin, empowering you to stand up to the immense pressures that big institutions, experts, and your peers—colleagues, friends, and family members—exert by urging you to use harmful skincare. Astonishingly, after several decades of trailblazing scientific discovery, most do not have a good grasp of their basic skin needs, fueling an explosion of damaging skincare practices and generically prescribed products. In short, most of us neither speak *Skinese* nor know how to properly care for our skin. We'll expose what's wrong with current popular ideas about skin, then provide a straightforward narrative for understanding your skin, answering its basic needs simply, concisely, and economically. You will learn to speak *Skinese*.

The origins of this book go all the way back to my childhood experiences as I'll explain shortly, leading to practicing bad skincare for years, which I turned around completely after having worked with tens of thousands of patients as a seasoned board-certified dermatologist.

Many of us assume that skincare is a simple and straightforward matter while the never-ending stream of "breakthroughs," products, and skincare routines stand in contrast to this assumption. Many, especially those suffering from chronic skin conditions or sensitive skin, may wonder: "If skincare is, indeed, simple, why the need for countless products and elaborate practices that don't work?" This book answers these questions — and more.

It's interesting to note that the source of most skincare information and skin products is the *skincare industrial complex* or *SIC*. The SIC, which I'll describe in more detail in Chapter 1, is made up of the giant skincare corporations, as well as many smaller companies, all of which are interconnected with skincare professionals who use and promote skincare products. While the SIC is not a monolith, there are recurring themes and attitudes that are pervasive throughout the industry, which is why I use the shorthand "The SIC" throughout the book. When appropriate, I'll give specific examples to illustrate a point. Understanding the SIC makes sense of contemporary skin grooming culture and can ultimately lead you to sensible and personalized skincare.

The SIC uses the common misconception of the power of modern science to push its agenda. Modern science is miraculous, having generated tremendous progress over the past century in understanding biology. Modern science possesses powerful tools such as biochemistry, genomics, proteomics, and engineering, making research much more robust and cheaper. While modern science and technological progress are amazing, the workings of the human body, including skin, are dizzyingly complex, so much so, I believe no amount of research or human insight could ever fully decipher it, let alone fully and reliably predict its behavior. Research will uncover more, but we can never see the entire picture or fully grasp the intricacy of skin. I do not want to discount the role of science in forming a more concrete understanding of biology or development of new technologies to improve human health.

Quite the opposite; I wholeheartedly support scientific research and appreciate the benefits it provides. However, with great power comes great responsibility in honestly and humbly recognizing our limitations, taking care not to overstep and rush to application of new discoveries and technologies without due diligence.

To properly care for skin, we must take a more abstract, intentional approach understanding it through basic reasoning.

In contrast, commonplace recommendations, "systems," "solutions," and pervasive attitudes miss the mark on several counts. They are unnecessarily and arrogantly complicated, often internally contradictory, and as such, lacking a clear direction. For example, a morning routine can incorporate a cleanser, a scrub, and a brush, all of which are abrasives that irritate the skin, rendering it drier, followed by application of a moisturizing sunblock, to supposedly address the dryness. Fireman arson much? Skincare culture is a mess.

Contemporary culture has devalued wisdom, i.e., applicable sensibility, in favor of "education," the curation and arbitrary use of information often dismissing good judgment. This is a mistake. Wisdom is timeless. Much of what is categorized as *information* is constantly changing, giving way to new claims. Education without wisdom is tantamount to prideful foolishness. Root your skincare in wisdom. Develop an unshakable and deep relationship with your skin, continuously assessing your *unique* needs, as this book will teach you. Straying from the principles outlined here will rob you of time, money, or worse: your physical, mental, and spiritual wellbeing.

While the skin is an unimaginably sophisticated organ, care for it is usually simple, if the skin is truly heard and understood. It's easy to get lost in the "science," the "studies," and "expert advice." For example, it's tempting to take the advice of a well-known veteran skincare professional, who shall remain nameless, starting her morning routine by "cleansing" with a "foaming gel" and following it up with a toner, claiming: "This neutralizes my skin's pH," which is nonsensical and factually incorrect. While this may seem harsh, both steps are unnecessary. Moreover, skin pH is neither neutral nor is it easily measurable outside the lab setting. The SIC added "scientific metric" purposefully for credibility.

Before we dive deeper into the SIC and its shenanigans, take a front seat into my personal skincare evolution. Here's a little of my background from me to you.

The Humble Beginnings of This Book

Obviously, I wasn't born a dermatologist or a skincare expert. Far from it. I come from humble skincare beginnings. I didn't have a routine while growing up, even though I did do some things consistently. Sort of. As a young boy, I used little soap and showered once a day. This was normal back in 1980's Israel, where I was born and raised. No one I knew showered more than once a day. There wasn't much pressure to use soap. Don't get me wrong. We used soap, shampoo, and even conditioner, known in Israel as hair softener. But I don't recall any special direction, method, or much discussion about it. I soaped whatever felt dirty. Shampooing was a toss-up. I didn't truly understand what a conditioner does[1] but used it occasionally, too. Cleaning, cleansing, exfoliating, scrubbing, disinfecting, moisturizing, conditioning, or *deep conditioning* wouldn't have meant anything to me, any kid I knew, and likely most adults.

In 1987, my dad moved our family to Canada where we lived for two years, returning to Israel thereafter. I was thirteen at the time, quickly realizing Canadian boys and girls were obsessing with something called body odor or BO. I had never heard of BO. My peers quickly brought me up to speed, anxiously, incessantly probing how many times a day I showered and whether I used soap and deodorant. Yeah, I know. Creepy. Teenagers are weird. Full disclosure: I did not use deodorant at the time the probing started. And yes, maybe those kids badgering me about BO were doing me a favor, nudging me into the fold of rose-smelling polite society. I wasn't alone. Everyone seemed to be dishing out and receiving the same treatment on occasion.

Sure enough, I started showering once, twice sometimes even three times a day, always using soap (the more fragrant the better) from head to toe, shampooing, conditioning, deodorant, the works. To be fair to my Canadian classmates, we were entering puberty, when the body starts producing distinctly adult, more pungent odors. However, the obsession with all things BO and skin grooming was pervasive, affecting all age groups, including younger children, as early as kindergarten, as my younger brother quickly found out.

In hindsight, Canadian kids ushered me into a religion of sorts. What were my considerations for forming those habits and joining the *movement*? Fitting in. Skin wellbeing was never a primary consideration. Without even knowing it, though, I slid into what I later termed the cult of skincare, complete with a catechism-like narrative and fundamental rituals in the name of social acceptance.

How did my Canadian counterparts develop such a pervasive and deeply rooted obsession with skincare? And, besides my being a stinky wild animal, why was I neither aware of most rituals nor treat them as sacraments prior to Canada? What was the difference between Israeli culture and North American culture, creating this religious rift?

"Americans love television. They wean their kids on it."
-Damon Killian, The Running Man (1987)

In a word: media. I had never seen anything like North American television prior to moving to Canada. Surely, countless immigrants and tourists prior to the spread of internet and expansion of telecommunications across the globe of the past 20 years share my sentiment. I vividly remember my first experience watching Canadian and American television; the variety, the fun, round the clock programming with something for virtually anyone. Besides seemingly endless choices, there was another feature distinct from Israeli television: commercials, i.e., mini promotional stories interrupting the main program, which I thought were just as engaging or even more fun than the full-length show. Crazy, I know. They were works of art.

To clarify, there was only one television channel in 1980's Israel, taxpayer-funded, government-operated, and mostly advertisement-free. Commercial television, unleashed in Israel in the early 1990s, remarkably transformed the country. In contrast, North American television, a largely private enterprise since its inception in the 1920s, has always received funds through paid advertisements just as it was with the radio. Vying for viewers' attention, television and commercial production must be exceptionally innovative, continuously evolving.

Exposure to commercially powered American and Canadian television clarified things regarding BO and more. Sweaty, stinky armpits as well as other cleanliness and hygiene issues could turn one into a social reject. Just kidding, but not at all. Cue the music. If you don't shut up, obey, shampoo, cleanse, exfoliate, and deodorize, the herd will expel you, friendless and sexless.

While many commercials were fun, cheeky, and clever, they were, in their own smiley, pleasant way, imposing and *totalitarian*. They were incisively directing, programming viewers to follow an all-immersive narrative to impeccable skin, silky hair, rosy BO, minty breath, and a perfect youthful life, little bits of upbeat utopian propaganda. The world consistently painted in skincare commercials goes beyond the adage of "sex sells," worshipping adolescence and folly. "Buy and use our product! All the cool kids are doing it! Or else..." It's emotionalism, appealing to the most basic human urges: feeling good about oneself instantaneously, becoming noticed, liked, and accepted.

So, media and downstream culture molding are tools at the SIC's disposal, promoting its prescriptions, leading to a big perennial payday. How do they do it and more importantly, how do they get away with it? We'll discuss this in detail in chapters I through IV. Before delving into the SIC and other players, let's set the stage for what's in this book.

What This Book Is Not

This book is neither a guide to becoming a dermatologist, nor does it certify you to give expert advice to others. Training as a dermatologist is a labor-intensive task of epic proportions taking many long years of exposure to the right mentors, working with colleagues, and countless patient encounters. For any of you reading this book who have seriously trained in any profession, you must know what it takes to achieve mastery in your respective area of expertise. Medicine, including dermatology, ideally requires deep understanding of the human body, healing, sciences, psychology, management, etc.

It's tough, taking immense dedication and perseverance. I am sincerely in awe of all dermatologists I've met over the years, even the ones I fundamentally disagree with. I recommend forging a relationship with a trustworthy dermatologist, who can guide you through issues and questions beyond the scope of basic skincare. As you'll find out, there is plenty you can do before seeking the advice of a professional.

What's in This Book?

First, we'll examine what is wrong with contemporary skincare, taking a deep dive into the belly of the SIC beast, a massive multilayered machine producing, promoting, and benefiting from the sale of skincare products, practices, and routines, many of which are useless and/or harmful.

Then, we critically evaluate a variety of SIC-sanctioned fallacies, misconceptions, and recommendations, many achieving norm status, forming the skincare matrix.

Next, we'll discuss how a mixture of tunnel-visioned good intentions, arrogance, and greed have led to tectonic shifts in skincare with a tsunami of consequences, most of which are still unknown. You'll see how moral panic the SIC promotes has affected human health, specifically, the disinfection craze or "The Great Dysbiosis" movement and the "War on the Sun" or "Sun Avoidance" movement. The disinfection craze has led to a widespread obsession with clearly harmful practices, altering skin integrity and the microbiome with unknown consequences, adding little to no value.

The sun avoidance movement, going strong for over 40 years, has promoted categorical demonization of sunlight in the name of cancer prevention, often turning a willful blind eye to the many overwhelming benefits of moderate sun exposure, which must be individually determined. This crusade ignores or minimizes individual needs for sun exposure (based on one's skin type and geographic location, for example), vulnerability to sun damage, as well as personal life circumstances dictating sun exposure. Additionally, the sun avoidance movement has encouraged using products whose true consequences for human health and biology are unknown.

Also, we look at the microbiome, which the SIC largely ignores or takes for granted, with unknown, yet potentially devastating costs. I reference the microbiome frequently in this book as a cautionary tale.

Finally, you can learn how to truly understand your skin using intuitive, simple, sensible terms. When you learn to speak *Skinese*, you can care for your skin intentionally, affordably, and effectively.

The Core Promises of This Book

A clear no-nonsense approach to skin. Through this book, you can develop a clear understanding of the SIC, and more importantly, a better approach to your own skin.

Rules for thee are the same for me. I practice what I preach, using all the appropriate skincare advice in this book, meaning everything except makeup tips. Hundreds, sometimes thousands of patients, friends, family, and skincare professionals have tried these recommendations with overwhelmingly positive feedback. Many were often initially skeptical. Some of you will smile remembering one of your elders, perhaps a grandparent, whose sensibility you may have dismissed as "old school."

Incalculable benefit. My recommendations will save you time and money that you can spend as you please. Time wasted on skincare could amount to over 2.5 years(!) of your life, as well as tens or even hundreds of thousands of dollars. But the greatest benefit of this book is better skin — in sickness and in health.

A permanent bullet-proof nonsense detector. You can develop well-founded confidence, knowing when someone is selling you propaganda, which is most skincare. While it's challenging even after realizing the game, you're free to choose, despite fear of missing out (FOMO) and other pressures.

When this book cannot help you any further, I will recommend a personalized evaluation by the best. We know the limitations of any medium or tool are necessary, so we don't abuse them. This book provides a comprehensive approach to caring for your skin. There are many issues beyond *basic* care requiring further expert evaluation and management. I'll let you know when we reach those limits, recommending seeing a dermatologist, sparing you from spinning your wheels, and inadvertently harming yourself or those under your care. Now, I'd like to introduce you to the church itself. Meet the industry, the *machine* making it all possible, as well as other players.

Chapter 1: Meet the Players

Meet the Skincare Industrial Complex or the SIC, an ever-expanding behemoth. The SIC is made up of large multinational multi-billion-dollar corporations, such as Procter & Gamble Co. (P&G), Unilever Group, L'Oreal S.A., and smaller companies all producing and promoting skincare products — creams, lotions, balms, serums, toners, sunblock, makeup removers, soaps, cleansers, shampoos, conditioners, scrubs, exfoliants, brushes, loofas, jade rollers... a seemingly endless skincare group.

The SIC also involves and uses skincare professionals including hairdressers, stylists, manicurists, cosmeticians, physician assistants, nurse practitioners, and physicians, i.e., dermatologists, as well as other fields, such as plastic surgeons, pediatricians, internists, and family doctors. All those professionals, most of whom the skincare-producing corporations do not employ, promote skincare products and practices that benefit the SIC. To be fair, some of the promoted products can be beneficial for the user or are at least something the customer/patient would have used anyway, so why not recommend something an expert endorses? I get it.

Promotion of products and skin grooming practices by the skincare professional class is complex ethically and morally. For one, this is not mere promotion, but also a glossing over or a legitimization of skincare products by virtue of professional expertise and prestige. As we'll see, most products are redundant, and many are harmful. By association with brand names responsible for useless products, skincare professionals, mostly unwittingly, whitewash those products and lend their credibility to support claims skincare corporations make.

Skincare professionals have a fiduciary relationship to their clients or patients, adding another layer of respectability and credibility to their endorsements.

Most do promotional work for little or no pay. Granted, there are some fringe benefits like complimentary products and treatments (mostly worthless or harmful). The return on this meager investment for corporations is priceless, considering the ripple effect of recommendations skincare professionals make to clients and patients, paying them forward to friends, family, even perfect strangers. So, many clients and patients of skincare professionals become another extension of the SIC, unwittingly incorporated into the promotional effort, paying for the privilege of promoting the products they use.

As mentioned earlier, I observed a stark cultural abyss between Israel and North America in the 1980s with regard to grooming and skincare. The one factor driving the North American skincare craze is digital media: commercial television and, increasingly, social media. We'll look at all those elements in detail in the coming chapters. Now, let's examine an underappreciated and recently defined element of the human body: the microbiome.

The microbiome consists of the microbial population living on and inside our bodies, composed of bacteria, fungi, viruses, protozoa, and even mites. Some of you may be thinking: these sound like dangerous categories of microbes and it's justified to get rid of them. That's a fair statement. However, it turns out this is not a black and white picture, but rather many organisms belonging to these groups live on our skin harmoniously, peacefully, and possibly fulfilling roles that we don't fully comprehend. The microbiome, particularly as an entity of value and specific roles, is a recent concept to the scientific community, spanning only a few decades. The microbiome inhabits not just the upper respiratory system, the gastrointestinal tract, the skin, etc. This is an incredibly complex phenomenon, varying from person to person, body part to body part, constantly changing. Its recent conceptualization, along with its mind-boggling complexity[2] exemplify the difficulty in studying and understanding the microbiome.

As scientists uncover more about the microbiome, it is clear how little we know and understand about its importance, appearing to extend beyond the tissue or area of the body it inhabits. While skin microbes are involved in regulating metabolism, inflammation, as well as microbial growth itself, scientists have linked the microbiome with neurological, cardiovascular, and endocrinological health, among other systems. While still a fairly obscure mode of therapy, fecal matter transplant (FMT) which is a deliberate alteration to one's microbiome, is gaining increasing attention, and potential applications[3,4].

I am convinced the microbiome is one of the greatest, most intriguing discoveries, and significant oversights of our time. Microbiomes can teach many lessons, even before much about them is known.

First, the microbiome (with the little we do know), is an irrefutable example of the complexity of biology. Second, with easy access and mostly unknown effects on the microbiome by skincare products and practices, the message is clear: Tread lightly. This is literally a part of our body easily accessible, highly susceptible to mutation and change, with unintended, unknown consequences. Third, the microbiome is an allegory for human arrogance and ingenuity used without temperance. The existence of the microbiome, its infinite complexity, and its vulnerability raise the possibility of other important microbiome-like phenomena.

Our understanding of the complex effects of skincare on the microbiome is virtually nonexistent. Theoretically, skincare may be responsible for such massive shifts in microbial populations, which are impossible to fully comprehend. If skincare products indeed affect the microbiome, then the effects are exponential, contagiously extending well beyond self-care. Self-applied skincare is the obvious way to affect the microbiome. As social creatures, human beings affect each other's skincare habits by passing on recommendations to significant others, acquaintances, and others. Mothers significantly affect their children's microbiome, providing the initial seed with placental transfer, birth canal, then skin to skin contact. This is a complex vertically transmitted inheritance. Furthermore, human beings seed each other horizontally, through direct touch, microbial cloud (see Chapter 4: A Look at Cleansing) or indirect contact with colonized fomites[5], mutually affecting the microbiome in numerous ways, with impossibly complex ripple effects.

Before looking at a few studies showing the effects of skincare products and ingredients, I'd like to make an important and seldom mentioned observation. Science and technology are restricted. Despite tools considered science fiction until recently, e.g., mass scale genotyping, bulk biochemical assays, and improved cell culture methods, there are still inescapable limitations.

With the ever-shifting biological complexity, data points sampled, location or space, methods used, investigator insight, not to mention second-hand layman interpretation of the reported results, encumber the intricacy and resolution of any assay or computer simulation. In other words, we are constrained by logistics, interpretation, and a limited predictive power. Even if we could piece together the behavior of a biological system in complete detail, we would still have to contend with future behavior remaining unpredictable. The rabbit hole simply goes too deep when it comes to the microbiome. Let's look at some evidence regarding skincare and its influence on the microbiome.

In a recent paper, Carlo Castillo and his colleagues[6] evaluated the effects of multiple skincare products and individual ingredients on a microbiome in culture, a mouse model, and healthy volunteers. The researchers discovered that many products and ingredients affect the microbiome, some of which are *not* antibacterial, or previously known to affect microbiology, demonstrating how little we know about the consequences of skincare product application. This study further highlights the fallacy arising in arbitrarily categorizing chemicals by a single industrial application whether it's fragrance, emulsifiers, or antibiotics, leading to erroneously assuming this is their *only* function.

This is just the tip of iceberg, and any ingredient can have multiple functions. This study, while detailed and ambitious, had logistical limits, *as any study does*. Two examples showing the constraints of this cutting-edge project are the number of human volunteers studied (six) as opposed to the billions of people, and the bacterial species analyzed (four) as opposed to hundreds if not thousands of different species found in skin, not to mention other microbes: protozoa, fungi, viruses, etc. Even on a superficial level the influence of skincare products and their ingredients appears profound.

Dr. Ian Myles and his colleagues[7] showed improvement of atopic dermatitis (AD) after seeding the skin of patients suffering from this condition[8] with a bacterium named *Roseomonas mucosa* (R. mucosa) harvested from healthy volunteers. When isolated from AD patients, R. mucosa worsened outcomes in a cell culture and mouse model, pointing to clear functional differences despite virtually appearing identical even by virtue of genomic assays.

This study shows how important even a single element of the microbiome can be in making a difference between normal and diseased skin. More so, the clear functional difference between *R. mucosa* sourced from healthy volunteers and AD patients, despite being biochemically indistinguishable is an example of the technological limitations of scientific inquiry.

Wang and colleagues[9] examined the effects of five cosmetic preservatives on bacteria isolated from the facial skin of fourteen healthy adults. The investigators found all five preservatives—methylisothiazolinone, iodopropynyl butylcarbamate, ethylhexylglycerin, methylparaben, and phenoxyethanol—inhibited the growth of resident microbiome when tested at the regulatory-allowed limit. The study was limited in several ways: the number of volunteers, the number of bacterial species tested, the methods used to test the effects of preservatives on microbiome, and so on.

The microbiome is therefore an awesome demonstration of our ignorance. Simply considering the inadvertent effect a woman's skincare could have on her microbiome health, the health of her children, and possibly other family members can be overwhelming. Yet, the SIC persistently promotes products through sophisticated propaganda with little consideration of those concerns.

Chapter 2: The Myth of Skintopia: The Perfect Skin

Does following the SIC lead to perfect skin? The holy grail of skincare, perfect skin, simply *does not exist*. It is a legend the SIC cultivates and promotes, propagating FOMO, promoting purchasing, and using products. But what about the models in media ads? Those models, handpicked out of thousands, get made up, airbrushed, and Photoshopped. Do not let them fool you. This is neither real nor is it a look anyone should strive for.

The staggering amount of skincare products whose claimed benefits are a stupefying array of variations of perfect skin are a testament to this falsehood. No amount of those products will make your skin perfect, even as they keep multiplying and the phrasing of the promise keeps changing.

So, skincare products do not make your skin perfect. Got it. How about improving skin? No, not really. Much like the promise of perfection, the ever-growing staggering number of products is a practical admission of their futility. If skincare leads to improvements, it sure takes a lot of effort and money to get there.

Regardless of truth in their advertising, this approach worked well for corporations promoting the perfect skin/life utopia. Employing psychological manipulation by shaming or guilting women, men, and children, the SIC has effectively permeated human behavior throughout the world. This affects the way people care for their own skin as well as their children's.

Parents, persuaded by the SIC narrative, pass it on to their children. Over the years, I've counseled thousands of well-meaning parents to back away from soaping and scrubbing their children in hot water and soap from head to toe. They clearly wanted to be the best parents possible, keeping their kids clean and safe. The SIC narrative is so seductive, it has successfully propagated as an idea contagion, a mind virus, or a prion affecting a critical mass, significantly influencing the way we spend staggering amounts of time, money, and other resources. This is big business.

The SIC keeps growing at an extraordinary rate. Between 2012 to 2020, the global skincare market grew from 99.6 billion to 148.3 billion and may reach 189.3 billion by 2025[10], clearly occupying a significant and steadily increasing share of people's lives, as if by compounding interest.

Skincare as You Know It Is a Giant Waste

I estimate over 90 percent of skincare and beauty products are redundant and potentially harmful, while the handful of helpful products are mostly misused, underused, overused, and abused. Complicating matters, recommendations, and general notions on the use of products result in skin damage, creating a need for other products. Fireman arson is a recurring SIC theme with consumers spending time, money, and other precious resources acquiring and using skincare products, and dealing with the consequences further compounds the issue.

This amounts to an incalculable expense countless women incur, as well as increasing numbers of men. The list includes but is not limited to the retail purchase cost of products, time spent using products, time spent dealing with side effects skincare products create (some companies promote adverse effects as *benefits*), purchase cost of secondary products addressing side effects of the primary products, disruption of personal and professional life due to skincare routine or side effects, clinic visits, prescription medications to address side effects, etc.

Many women report using the following: a gentle cleanser in the morning, a scrub, a face brush, a washcloth, a moisturizing cream or lotion, concealer, eyeliner, moisturizing soap or body wash in the shower, a loofa/body brush, a moisturizing shampoo, a conditioner, a makeup remover, a face serum, and an eye cream. This long list costs anywhere from hundreds to thousands of dollars or more annually. I know you may be thinking, "This guy doesn't get what pressures I am dealing with to get my skin to look great." As the book progresses, we'll examine how to deal with those pressures much more effectively and affordably. According to some estimates, the average cost of skincare for an American woman over a lifetime exceeds $225,000.[11]

I've heard plenty of versions of the reasoning behind such a stunning squandering of time, money, and health. At the root of all of this is the common human need to improve or maintain physical appearance, by investing in one's skin, hair, and nails. $225,000 is a conservative figure, only factoring in the mere retail cost of various skincare products. This figure did not account for the time spent on applying skincare products, which one survey estimated to be an average of 55 minutes a day for an adult woman[12] or roughly 335 hours or two weeks a year. If the average life expectancy for a woman in the United States is 81.4 years and she practices skincare from age 15, she may spend over *two and half* (!) years of her life on skincare application.

Skincare is fortified by a strong set of beliefs in the value of these practices to promote healthy skin. Sure enough, some products contribute to short-term improvement in skin appearance or the immediate way the skin feels. For example, you can get "glow" by either adding oils and surfactants to certain products, or abrasive elements, such as microbeads. Countless skincare products create a short-term, unsustainable improved appearance effect, often leading to persistent damage. Rinse, recycle, repeat. The effects of skincare beyond this superficial impression are largely unknown, meaning largely unexplored, undetermined, their magnitude, their extent is unimaginable and largely incomprehensible, beyond the grasp of science as a limited method.

In the short and intermediate timeframes, many skincare products create visible and palpable undesired effects. Specifically, easily noticeable skin drying, abrasion, irritation, and injury. Any tightness, itch, burning you may be feeling after using a skincare product or device is a sign of irritation and disruption of skin integrity. Redness, glow, as well as widespread textural changes are all visible signs of irritation and changes in skin biology. Changes are often temporary and reversed by normally functioning skin.

The changes persist when the skin can no longer reverse environmental damage on its own, for a variety of reasons. This is where people run into trouble and experience persistence of symptoms generally associated with improvement, i.e., tightness, burning, redness, as well as other hallmarks of freshness. Whether it's insufficient production of protective elements such as oils, persistent inflammation as in the example of rosacea, microbial overgrowth, or any combination of those phenomena. So-called sensitive skin reaches a critical threshold. Once someone crosses this line, the skin cannot reverse course, and irritation persists. In those cases, consultation with a dermatologist can be the beginning of the solution. But even with the best of intentions, expertise and recommendations, people can derail their own healing.

Old habits die hard. I frequently advise patients their practices are the root of the problem only to listen to doubt and hear on follow-up visits they "had to cleanse a little bit..." with the problem persisting, or even worsening. This is essentially a religious battle. Abandoning skincare is challenging, much like a deeply held religious belief or an addiction.

How does the SIC achieve this level of loyalty in its numerous devotees? By promoting strong beliefs about skincare, subsequently driving behavior, namely the religious rites of the skincare routine. Many of those convictions are false. Let's examine some common assumptions and assertions regarding the SIC and skincare.

Skincare Fallacies and Superstitions

"Skin (Hair, Nails) Is Dead Tissue"

Whether consciously or unconsciously, countless people regard their skin, hair, and nails as "dead tissue." This is one of the justifications for the cavalier and careless ways with which people treat their skin, figuratively blow-torching it. This is a misconception. The skin, hair, and nails are absolutely not dead tissue.

First, there is the microbiome, comprised of countless living organisms coexisting with skin, hair, and nails. Second, skin cells, namely keratinocytes, are alive, undergoing an intentional cell death,[13] fortifying the skin through cornification, formation of keratin[14]. This highly complex process is by design: "dead keratinocytes" are necessary for maintaining skin integrity, among other functions. So, considering skin a dead tissue, implying it's redundant is nonsensical. The skin is not dead, and even in their so-called death process, skin cells continue carrying out essential functions, many of which are beyond our understanding.

The "Trusted Brand" Fallacy

"Trusted brand" is a word game designed to increase consumer confidence in a single product, a product line, or even a whole corporation. Associating with a dermatologist, another skincare professional, an actor portraying a skincare professional, or citing statistics promotes credibility, and ultimately sales. This is a fallacy on several levels. First, the definition of "trusted" is unclear. What is a trusted brand, who trusts and to do what exactly is open to interpretation. Second, what part of a brand gets the trust? Is it one product, two products, or all of them? In short, this fallacy is a promotional tool creating an image of nebulous health benefits for the advertised subject. An extension of this concept is the "dermatologist trusted" or "dermatologist recommended."

The "Dermatologist Recommended" Fallacy

This is an iteration of the trusted brand fallacy, promoting nonsensical credibility. One's ability to recommend anything wholesale is ridiculously limited. With a few rare exceptions, the applicability of one dermatologist's experience to the end user is meaningless; a product working marvelously for one person does not apply to everyone. A dermatologist making a recommendation in a clinic ideally considers a staggering number of variables. Making a personally tailored recommendation takes years of experience with thousands of patients, which stands in contradiction to the slogans or friendly faces staring at you from product packaging or promotional materials. There's no interaction, evaluation, or personal considerations.

The "Dermatologist Routine" Fallacy

This concept has exploded with the growing popularity of social media, with dermatologists or other skincare professionals of various credentials and repute sharing their personal daily product application rituals. The genre is rife with rationalization, axiomatic doctrine of the "good for the skin" ilk, references to specific brand names, and highly technical descriptions, with several inherent problems. First, despite the best of intentions, most so-called routines are not beneficial. Many promote abrasion, compensatory or mindless moisturization, with a sprinkle of snake oil and sunblock. Second, whether this works for the influencer or not has nothing to do with an audience that has different skin characteristics and needs. Third, shared routines are fleeting, easily shifting for the promoter as one's skin changes. In reality, there is *no such thing as a skincare routine*; people's needs are everchanging.

The "Everybody" Fallacies

Many promote skincare products and practices as universally necessary and beneficial. If you've engaged in discussion of skincare with professionals or frequent skincare users, you've likely heard an assertion like "everybody needs to moisturize." Skincare is personal, and the individual must therefore not follow generalizations such as "everyone" or "everybody.

The one exception to generalizing prescriptions regarding skincare is: Everyone *should* get to know their own skin and understand its needs. Cultivating this fundamental skill is at the root of any meaningful and sustainable skincare. Let's look at some of those generalizing fallacies.

The "Everybody Needs to Moisturize" Fallacy

I've encountered this assertion countless times while counseling patients in the clinic and seen it on numerous resources online. "Everybody needs to moisturize." The reality is far more nuanced and must be determined on a case-by-case basis. Not everybody, not even most people need to moisturize. Moisturization is for people with dry and sensitive skin and unnecessary for normal or oily skin.

Moisturization is one of the most misunderstood concepts as well as one of the most frequently promoted practices in skincare. In my experience, the world largely divides into people who do not moisturize and those who moisturize arbitrarily regardless of need. Neither is correct. We'll examine moisturizing in more detail as we progress through the book, ultimately getting to sensible real-world guidelines.

The "Everybody Needs to Use Sunblock" Fallacy

In the American Academy of Dermatology (AAD) Sunscreen FAQS, in response to "Who needs sunscreen?" the answer is: "Everyone..." This is a false assertion. Skincare is an individual pursuit as every person's skin needs are unique. Not everyone tans, burns, derives the same benefits, or suffers the same damage from sun exposure. Generalizing statements paint "everyone" into the same corner, as if their skin-sunlight relationship and skin responses are the same. We'll discuss this further in Chapter 10.

The "All Moisturizers Are the Same" Fallacy

To the unsuspecting consumer there is little indication of any distinction between different moisturizers: lotions, creams, ointments, or balms. This is a fallacy. Moisturizing or adding and sustaining water content on the skin is a highly complex matter, achievable by an occlusive, a humectant, or both. Occlusives are oils providing a waterproof layer over the skin. Humectants attract water to the skin, whether it's from outside or within the body. Moisturizing depends on specific properties of the ingredients of the product, as well as its application.

The more a product is water-based, like lotions and creams, the less occlusive it can be. So, lotions and creams are generally ineffective occlusives compared with ointments or balms. Not only are water-based lotions and creams poorly occlusive, but some of their ingredients, specifically emulsifiers, can increase skin permeability, leading to trans-epidermal water loss (TEWL).

We'll get back to a clear prescription for the use of moisturizers a little later.

The Cleansing Fallacy

Countless times I've asked people to stop using detergents or synthetic detergent alternatives on their skins only to hear a gasp, followed by the eternal question "...but what about the dirt?"

Unless you rolled around in actual dirt, soil, cow manure, whatever, your skin is not dirty. Whatever *dirt* is, it's a combination of detachable skin cells, also known as "dander," microbes and various compounds, the skin and its resident microbiome produce. When lifted off the skin physically or chemically, those elements can undergo oxidation, appearing brown or black. Sound familiar? So, while parts of the skin appear as dirt once removed from the skin, they are not dirt. Categorizing the upper layers of the skin as dirt contributes to the wild abandon we tend to use to treat skin.

Despite remarkable scientific developments in understanding the components of the skin, skin architecture, and an increasing awareness of the importance of the microbiome[15], we are nowhere near understanding the full complexity and marvel of skin biology.

Regarding "cleaning" itself, first, as definitions go, it is impossible to pin down exactly what a person is supposed to clean. However, the result of any "cleaning" practices is diluting, thinning, stripping, or otherwise washing away elements naturally found on the skin's surface. Interestingly, try as you may, you will not find any convincing evidence supporting the benefits of the extensive practices or "routines" the SIC promotes to address "dirt." The consequences of any cleansing practice, even if well tolerated, are alteration and disruption of the upper layers of the skin, physically, chemically, and biologically. This may seem like a small thing, especially if you're not sensing any immediate changes. The seldom acknowledged truth is we don't know the full effects of "cleaning" or "removing dirt."

The "Gentle" Cleansing Fallacy

In the beginning of cleansing, there was water. Water is the most common and oldest "cleanser" of skin and can decrease bacterial counts on the skin[16] as well as increase TEWL[17]. You read it right. Washing with water alone can decrease bacterial numbers on skin as well as disrupt the skin barrier. No soap needed. The old ritual of handwashing before meals or other water-based cleansing traditions makes microbiological sense.

Adding soaps, naturally occurring fatty acid salts or synthetic detergents (syndets), enhances the effects of water. Why all the variations? Why create a so-called upgrade to soap in the form of syndets? Soap is harsh and can inflict significant damage. The solution: develop gentler synthetic detergents that are not as "damaging." Why not settle for water only, which is the least damaging of all the washing techniques?

In the case of handwashing to prevent the spread of infection or remove/ dilute unwanted grease, detergents, including soap, fare better than water and can be used for a maximal effect. Controlling body odor requires using detergents on armpits, groin, gluteal cleft or "butt-crack," and other skin folds, i.e., under pendulous breasts, or other body folds in the morbidly obese. That's it.

Putting aside the need to curb the spread of infection and the need to smell good, what about washing for "cleansing" the face, the arms, the legs, the face, or the scalp? The origins for "cleansing" recommendations are complex and longstanding, including societal trends that medical professionals clearly helped and SIC promotion fueled.

Let's take a close look at cleansing. Cleaning or cleansing promotes two major biological effects: first, lowering bacterial counts (likely more broadly on a pan microbial level, meaning fungi, viruses, protozoa, mites, etc.) and second, diluting or washing away functional elements of the skin barrier, including proteins, lipids, carbohydrates, ions and metals, bases, acids, etc.

Lowering microbial counts is a selling point due to the "disinfection craze." However, increasing skin permeability, as well as changing other properties in unknown ways is unappealing. Many would think twice before using a product known to disrupt skin integrity and increase TEWL, keeping this aspect out of SIC promotional campaigns. It goes against the narrative equating skincare with promotion of health. It doesn't look good.

Also cleansing increases the need for compensatory practices such as moisturizing. Who sells moisturizers? The SIC does. So, cleansing in all its forms, even the justified ones, creates a need for a second practice: moisturization, the products often sold by the same corporation, constituting a fireman arson. As seen in the following example, the SIC evolves and uses scientific discovery on more than one front.

According to its website, Gallinée Microbiome Skincare is "...the first beauty brand to care for your microbiome, from head to toe. The results? Strong, glowy, & rebalanced skin all around![18]" Inspection of their ingredient lists reveals run-of-the-mill "cleansing products": surfactants, preservatives, fragrance, and in some cases heat-inactivated lactobacilli, a common probiotic ingredient.

While this is an honorable idea, more data are necessary to prove their products benefit the microbiome. The studies included on the website have design limits, appearing open (no blinding), missing controls, and having few volunteers – only 22. More deficiencies in methodology are the length of the study, 21 days, and the subjective survey method asking for users' opinions about the effects of the product rather than measuring objective data. More so, it is impossible to judge what ingredient in the product is responsible for the positive effects the users reported, or whether they are objectively beneficial. In short, there is no quality evidence Gallinée's products have any benefit for the microbiome. Interestingly, Gallinée Microbiome Skincare has garnered investments from Unilever Ventures, a giant conglomerate of various brand names, many of which manufacture skin cleansing products, forming yet another fireman arson loop. See the antimicrobial fallacy.

So, whether it's an innocent good faith (albeit, misguided) attempt, a scam, or a combination of both, the SIC creates the need for moisturizing through promoting skin-damaging practices, laundered through language games, seductively and erroneously termed "cleansing." As we age and the skin becomes drier, and more sensitive, the ability to make up for the effects of "cleansing" diminishes, as do potential profits from the sales of moisturizers.

Shampoos represent another category of "cleansers" seeing a trend of adding adjectives attesting to the product's enhanced tolerability such as "gentle" or "moisturizing." Several different approaches launder this product's reputation. Companies can designate products gentle by making them free of compounds deemed harsh, such as sodium lauryl sulfate, while keeping other ingredients not yet fallen out of favor. Another way of making a product gentle is adding ingredients from the snake oil category, such as seaweed extract, plant extract, goat milk, etc. As we'll explore later, skincare snake oils are a broad category of ingredients with little to no evidence of health benefits used to create a buzz and increasing sales. Remember, nothing here is arbitrary or redundant. Or how about just calling the product gentle without changing anything? Much like the syndet category, the so-called gentling is meaningless since there is largely no need for shampooing in the first place. I know this is a shocking statement. More on that later.

Bottom line: The shifting of cleansing-speak is nothing more than an elaborate sleight of hand, offering less of what's unnecessary for starters. Moreso, it is knowingly doubling down on moot and possibly harmful recommendations with technological innovation and word games.

It's risky for a big corporation to disavow its longstanding money-making products and concepts. The impact could be as simple as revenue loss and possibly lead to legal ramifications. SIC corporations would much rather come up with technological or linguistic fixes: add new compounds, replace old ingredients with new ones, or change the descriptive language around the product incorporating terms like gentle or microbiome friendly.

There is no regulation or standard of what gentle or gentler means, making this language game utterly meaningless and easily manipulable.

The Baby Product Fallacy

Most parents are deeply concerned with the wellbeing of their kids, especially babies. Many go to great lengths to buy the best skincare products for their babies, creating a new generation of customers for the SIC. Sell parents on the safety and wellbeing of their babies, and you have a customer for life. So, it is no surprise the baby product market is highly lucrative, and the buzzword baby is synonymous with a high level of scrutiny and safety.

There are no laws regulating the labeling of products as baby products. Therefore, the use of the word baby to describe specialty products as safer is *meaningless*. One example is Johnson's Head-To-Toe Baby Wash and Shampoo. With the ingredient list containing fragrance as well as potential allergens (e.g., Cocamidopropyl betaine, Decyl glucoside; Lauryl glucoside) and irritants (e.g., Sodium cocoyl isethionate), this product is not provably safer for a baby than competing adult washing products. This is *not* a condemnation of the product itself but of the linguistic facelift by the arbitrary baby label. This trend is here to stay, meaning you are responsible for examining baby products with a critical eye. Whenever purchasing a baby product, ask yourself how is this product safer for a baby than other products on the market?

Baby Wipes

Baby wipes are a popular category of products, used by parents of babies and young children, as well as countless adults, seeking to treat their skin gently. Arbitrarily categorized for baby application, these products are largely sheets of various soft fibrous porous materials, soaked in liquid concoctions of ingredients declaratively making wiping easier and decreasing friction on the skin. However, many baby wipes have adulterations with ingredients posing a risk to skin health and integrity, specifically fragrance and preservatives. Even the very purest of baby wipes, i.e., the ones boasting the bare minimum of ingredients in their immersion solution, contain benzalkonium chloride, a preservative. Fragrance is there purely to enhance product experience, promoting repeat use. The reason for insistence on preservatives is the combination of water and wipes, easily serving as a microbial growth medium.

My advice is to avoid using baby wipes as much as possible. They are expensive and redundant vanity products. You are better off using a soft two- or three-ply toilet paper to minimize friction with wiping, or paper towels that you can dip in water as needed.

If you must use baby wipes, choose wisely with the least number of ingredients as possible.

If you develop redness, flakiness, itch, burning, or pain distinctly over the wiping area, assume this is related to your use of baby wipes and stop using them, switching to dry toilet paper.

The "Antimicrobial" Fallacy

The disinfection movement swept Western culture (and beyond) with a combination of technological innovation combined with nothing short of a mass hysteria/moral panic. More and more people automatically "disinfect" fomites and human skin, using products meant to kill microbes: antibacterial wipes, sprays, soaps, or sanitizers. Considering this crowd madness raises several points.

First, these practices target the microbiome, with virtually no clue as for what the downstream effects are. Second, except for very specific cases where infection control is important as in the healthcare or food industries, there is no benefit. In fact, there is likely much harm in disinfecting the environment, as well as the skin, including eliminating microbes that are important to human biology fulfilling various functions, underexposure of the immune system to microbes, antimicrobial resistance, making room for dangerous pathogens to take hold on the skin, diluting human-derived skin elements of unknown significance, as well as toxicity to human beings beyond disrupting the microbiome. Third, disinfection, "purification from infectious matter; the destruction of the contagium or germs of infectious diseases,"[19] doesn't truly disinfect, but rather briefly decreases numbers of microbes, altering microbial populations with regard to species diversity, genetics, and long-term function, in some ways indefinitely. Fourth, handwashing itself is of limited utility not eliminating all microbes on the skin and powerless to affect the microbial cloud surrounding each person.

The "Vitamin" Fallacy

Like the "everyone" fallacies, everyone accepts vitamins in both topical[20] and oral supplement forms as something simply good for everyone, irrelevant of one's personal circumstances or the mode of application/intake. As covered later, this categorical view of vitamins leads to misuse, including inappropriate consumption, underdosing, and worst of all, false and unmet hopes regarding the desired effects of supplements. This is especially egregious in categories such as hair loss, where even with the correct diagnosis and treatment it may take many months to turn things around or achieve a meaningful result. In every single case, I've counseled a patient taking hair supplements the bottom-line was the same. The patient was spending time and money taking unnecessary supplements, while their hair loss was either unchanged or worse.

The "Multivitamins" Fallacy

Tests have repeatedly shown multivitamin (MVI) combinations to be useless[21] and possibly even harmful with little public awareness[22]. The rationale behind MVI is to conveniently package many different compounds at quantities determined to be the daily requirements or necessary amount. Another way of packaging MVI is putting together a combination of ingredients under the claim of a specific benefit, e.g., hair supplements, nail supplements, or skin supplements. Sounds great, but let's look at the facts.

First, the supplement paradigm works assuming your diet is inadequate, while in the Western world there is no shortage of nutritious food. Whole food provides and should provide the daily requirements. So, unless you're truly deficient in some form of nutrient, a balanced diet of unprocessed whole foods widely available is all you need. Second, your daily requirement of anything is not a steady amount as storage levels and bodily utilization of any vitamin change day to day and from life period to life period, e.g., infanthood, early childhood, adolescence, young adulthood, pregnancy, etc. You could have all the iron you need one day and deficient the next due to blood loss.

The same quantity taken continuously is inadequate and cannot possibly be the daily requirement.

Third, the limited number of compounds in MVI cannot compete with the nuance and complexity of whole foods. Fourth, some of the forms of so-called vitamins and nutrients are not readily absorbable and are of virtually little or no value, e.g., zinc sulfate has poor absorption as opposed to zinc gluconate. Moreover, different vitamins and micronutrients require different conditions for absorption, so the value and absorption of MVI ingredients is uneven with wide variations.

Fifth, if you are truly deficient in a specific micronutrient, MVI would likely fall significantly short of your needs. No one size fits all and the supplement dose would depend on the severity of the deficiency, as well your ability to absorb and retain the nutrient in question. I always strive to establish an endpoint when the patient can stop taking the medicine or supplement. The goal of medicine is to help people live their lives as freely as possible, including freedom from unnecessary treatment.

So, it's clear the SIC relies on many false assertions to promote its prescriptions – products, practices, and the concept of what constitutes healthy skin. How does the SIC do this and more importantly how does it get away with it? In the next chapter we'll cover many ways in which the SIC can manipulate consumer opinion, belief, and practice.

Chapter 3:
How Does the SIC Manipulate Us and Get Away With It?

The SIC has mastered the art of branding, promotion, and maintenance. It mainly accomplishes this through manipulation of language, using words whose meaning has changed or even reversed, sharing your vocabulary but not your dictionary. There are many facets to this magic trick.

First, let's give the devil his due. The SIC provides valuable tools to billions of people: decreasing the spread of infection[23], improving presentability, promoting skin health, and promoting a sense they're doing something of value regardless of benefit. Second, the SIC is subject to virtually no government oversight. Third, the SIC has an *assumed* fiduciary responsibility with its customers with a high level of public trust. Public faith in the SIC is akin to institutional trust. Fourth, the SIC is innovative with regard to various aspects of human psychology, effectively putting this knowledge to good use whether it's product design, packaging, promotional campaigns, and so on. Fifth, our understanding of skin health and standards that we hold the SIC to are archaic and largely overlook the microbiome, metabolome, and more as significant elements of the skin.

The True Role of Skincare Products and Ingredients

To understand behavior, and its motivation, it's important to understand one's underlying needs. The SIC exists to make money through the sale of skincare products. Sounds simple enough, but there are various layers to this statement, and not all of them are on the up and up. Let's examine the composition of skincare products and see how their design and makeup boost corporate goals. What are some common corporate needs embodied by product properties? Prolonging shelf life, attracting customers through product physical appeal as well as promotional appeal, and retaining customers are a few. Meeting these goals means big bucks, especially with a multi-billion-dollar enterprise. Corporate needs take away from the value of the product as it translates to serving your skin needs or even worse, making the product potentially harmful.

Serving corporate needs is a costly proposition: money, time, and possible harm to your health. Try reading the ingredient list on the package of a favorite skincare product, looking up the purpose of each item. You'll quickly realize most of those ingredients are there to serve corporate needs, whether it's preservatives (including vitamin E, i.e., alpha tocopherol), emulsifiers, texturizers, stabilizers, fragrance, and snake oils.

Now, you may be asking, what's wrong with extending shelf life, making a product look better, more pleasant to apply or smelling nicer? The short answer: nothing. There is nothing inherently wrong with any of those goals. One could argue adding snake oil to skincare products is dishonest. But from the manufacturer's perspective, if consumers demand snake oil, they're bound to get those ingredients one way or another. It's unclear what is the chicken and what's the egg, i.e., using snake oil in products or public demand, likely being a bit of both.

Extending shelf life may work for you as well in case you're in the skincare hoarding business. But a long shelf life comes at a price – added preservatives or stabilizers. Most users consider preservatives used in skincare products to be safe, which *does not equal* safe. We assume things are a certain way based on heuristics, creating shortcuts, concluding a product and its components are safe. Preservatives, and other ingredients, have properties, many of which are unknown. On the macro level and in the short and intermediate timeframe, preservatives may irritate your skin. On the micro level, preservatives are antimicrobial, as well as molecular and product-consistency stabilizers, slowing down product decay. The micro effects of preservatives on skin are not well known, but it's evident these elements can and do affect the microbiome. At present, the volume of scientific research examining the issue is a few dozen papers, which is negligible.

Emulsifiers or surfactants are frequently used in creams, lotions, and other products. On the macro level they may sensitize the skin or irritate it. On a cellular and molecular level, emulsifiers can disrupt cell membranes, increase TEWL, etc. This means a component incorporated into a moisturizer may lead to losing moisture or altering skin pH, undermining the *declared* benefit of the product[24]. In addition, surfactants affect the microbiome, and their true long-term effects are unclear.

Dyes, used to color skincare products, are potential irritants and allergens, as are fragrances. As with preservatives, there are plenty of unknowns about their biochemical and microbiological effects. Interestingly, many dyes, such as gentian violet, brilliant green, and others used in clinical practice and over-the-counter, have antimicrobial effects. The status quo remains static by overlooking or dismissing the significance of those possibilities. The snake oil category is so broad and versatile it's impossible to collectively say what effects they would have on product cost, efficacy, safety, or harm.

What does "safe" really mean? Immediate and short-term skin reactions are the gold standard of safety. Irritation, allergenicity, and other visible localized mostly short-term reactions are a mere fraction of potential effects of skincare ingredients. They are an arbitrary gold standard because they occur over the application area, develop concurrently with product use, are clearly noticeable, and so relatively easy to connect with the product. With time and experience post product launch, new understandings of the effects of compounds expand. Some are mutagenic, some carcinogenic, some teratogenic, some will undoubtedly tie to effects on the microbiome and beyond the comprehension of contemporary science.

The ripple effect of any one of these possibilities is practically unimaginable. There are simply too many variables and many more unknowns to assess potential harm of most skincare products. We must take chances in life. As a matter of principle, this is reasonable. However, when it comes to most skincare products, it seems excessive so many people take so many chances on a collection of habits of such little proven benefit. The dearth of evidence for the benefit of most skincare practices has several aspects.

First, there is little interest in putting many of the assertions the SIC makes to rigorous well-designed scientific scrutiny by large, long-term, double-blind, randomized, controlled studies. Even if there was widespread interest and such studies existed, their value would have limits. Not everything can be meaningfully quantified and statistically analyzed. Even if a well-designed study shows significant benefit of a specific practice for a specific skin element, it will still fail to address every possible short- and long-term benefit and safety, as well as apply to every future user. This is not only impossible but also completely unnecessary with most skincare practices and ingredients addressing manufactured or made-up problems rather than real ones.

There are several ways in which skin needs or problems (and other health issues) do not exist. All these processes heavily rely on cavalier, careless assumptions, and generalizations regarding extremely complex phenomena. First is to focus on a problem, not yet existing, such as future aging or deterioration. Complexity aside, anyone's ability to predict how aging unfolds and address it has limits.

Second, the SIC is responsible for creating unrealistic expectations by photo manipulation, using the language of perfection and other forms of psychological influence to create an insecurity about one's self-image. Skin free of blemishes, moles, bumps, wrinkles, bruises, flakiness, and other noticeable imperfections does not exist, certainly not in perpetuity.

Third, beyond the standard of perfection, the SIC creates a superhuman standard, separate, and elevated from the perfection bar. This includes terms referring to skin appearance and personal image, such as glowing, radiant, and more. This promotes a new set of insecurities or unmet urgent and important expectations calling people to action.

Fourth, the SIC points out real skin phenomena such as flakiness or blemishing, which multiple inherently different processes can cause, and heavy-handedly lumps them together, thereby offering a categorical and generic solution under the pretense of individually tailored treatments. Flaky skin can form because of multiple causes, including but not limited to dryness[25,26], old age, irritant dermatitis, allergic contact dermatitis, psoriasis, seborrheic dermatitis, fungal infection, yeast overgrowth, scarring, etc. Any one of those conditions needs individual attention and often with great nuance to meaningfully improve. The wide array of available products creates the impression of a multitude of available solutions. However, the adequacy of any SIC product to provide a solution is not a given and in most cases is not granularly determined due to lack of deep understanding of the nature of the problem or the product's utility.

Fifth, another way of manufacturing a skin problem is to create a need for a certain way for the skin to feel and associating sensation with a positive buzzword, in line with the Pepsodent™ effect, which I'll discuss in more detail later in this chapter. This is distinct from improving skin conditions because in most cases conscious and persistent sensations over the skin are a sign of injury or disruption. Numerous campaigns have interlinked sensations created by irritation of the skin, like tightness, dryness, burning, and redness to buzzwords or slogans such as fresh, refreshed, wakeup call, creating a niche for detergents, scrubs, exfoliants, toners, other forms of abrasives, etc.

Sixth, emphasizing natural and common phenomena that can stigmatize, and difficult to self-detect such as BO, creates motivation and a niche for a variety of product categories, including cleansers, deodorants, antiperspirants, and perfumes.

Seventh, problematizing the natural features of the skin such as oils, bacteria, and other components helps create a need for whole classes of products: detergents, toners, antimicrobials, etc.

Looking Good or Feeling Good Does Not Equal Healthy

An interesting point is there is little evidence of the benefit of most products in those categories, while generating revenues in the billions. So, how do so many product categories with dubious benefit sell so well? Where's the public backlash or more simply abandonment? This is a complicated issue. Most people tolerate skincare products well. This does not mean skincare products are safe, but rather they appear to be associated with an acceptable profile of side effects within the inspected scope. Well-tolerated in the short run and according to arbitrary guidelines *does not equal* safe.

The challenge of verifying the safety of skincare products is a fool's errand. This begins with the fact most studies aim to observe adverse effects related to skin only, and there are limits of time and the study's scope. So, unless there are noticeable[27], widespread, and consistent or recurring side effects over the short period of time the company tests a product, a manufacturer may launch a product without additional scrutiny. This seems reasonable. After all, one can never truly cover all bases, and skincare manufacturing is a business first and foremost.

Standards for skincare recall address three major categories: contamination with infectious agents such as bacteria or yeast, toxins/irritants, and carcinogens. These categories all manifest as potential noticeable and tangible physical harm, whether it's infection, irritation, or cancer. Any recall over more obscure effects such as dysbiosis, or disruption of the microbiome, is not realistic or applicable at present. Large institutions such as government agencies are too cumbersome, as well as remarkably inefficient in formation and implementation of policy to keep up with new data or public opinion. Therefore, the ability of any large institution to protect public interest swiftly and decidedly is negligible. So, there is very little standing between you, the consumer, and the monopoly of the SIC.

What about animal testing? Ethics or morality aside, they do provide some degree of assurance on the way to human trials. There are several caveats to animal studies. First, animals and humans are different, and each species has a unique physiology, i.e., animal findings are not necessarily translatable to humans. Second, lab animals used in testing are usually clonal, meaning almost identical or very close genetically and phenotypically[28], certainly different for human populations with a wide genetic and phenotypic variability. The genetic uniformity of lab animal species can mask serious issues with the tested product. Third, regardless of how reliable lab animals are there are only so many ways to test an ingredient or a product, as well as limited time. Fourth, lab animals cannot communicate as people do, and so cannot give verbal feedback about their use experience. Testers cannot assess psychoactive, emotional, and extrasensory effects. No two people are the same.

The Wild West: the Fallacy of Government Oversight

Regulation of skincare products is a fool's errand. There are simply too many companies and brands for any government to get its tentacles around, coupled with a continuous and perpetual development of our understanding of biology and skin. Many governments can't help themselves and must do something. The result is the appearance of law and order, while in reality, anything goes.

In ways of regulating cosmetic products, there are various standards across the globe. Whether it's the United States government's Food and Drug Administration (FDA) or the European Union, there are clear guidelines in place to enforce some level of assumed safety of products. Those guidelines obviously rely on the available information regarding the biological effects of chemical ingredients. This information is always as good as the most recent observations, obviously evolving as our understanding of various compounds and their bioeffects becomes more apparent. Talcum is one example of such rolling regulation. Widely used for many years as a perfectly safe product, talcum is now associated with some forms of cancer. And while the evidence remains inconclusive, more research is necessary to further our understanding of talcum's safety.

Triclosan is an antibacterial compound. The FDA now bans once the darling of the SIC, as well as skincare professionals as a readily available antibacterial agent, for use in over-the-counter antiseptic wash products.

Parabens are a group of preservatives used in skincare, among other industries and many now consider them safe, including dermatologists[29]. The insistence on safety of parabens stems from the low incidence of undesired effects along the usual surveyed categories of contact allergy and "toxicity." Again, this claim of safety comes from interpretation of the existing evidence. While reports are scant as of 2023, some parabens clearly affect the microbiome[30]. Thus, claims of paraben safety refer to immediate observable effects whose infrequency is indisputable, rather than their largely unknown downstream effects.

The SIC's Deep Ties with Both Clinical and Academic Dermatologists Promote an Association Fallacy

The ties of cosmeceutical and cosmetic companies to actual healthcare providers and academic researchers are extensive. This ranges from medical assistants, managers, nurses, physician assistants and doctors on the clinical side as well as research assistants, graduate students, and principal investigators on the academic side. This relationship begins early in training and in school, including dermatology trainees or even medical students interested in dermatology.

The ties form through personal connections, through sales representatives providing free product samples, brand name merchandise (e.g., pens, track-pads, shirts, hats, nifty handbags, backpacks, umbrellas, or other items with the brand logo), food, or even funds in the way of research grants and other financial rewards. Most of this goes on with little to no linear transaction, i.e., no quid pro quo. For example, the doctor or researcher accepting the benefit does not immediately do anything for the representative or the corporation. And while the sentiment among healthcare providers varies from affection and indifference through resentment, disdain, disgust, or even hatred of these efforts, this massive campaign has been ongoing for many decades almost uninterrupted. The goal of this endeavor is clear: recruiting ambassadors, representatives, and promoters for brand names.

Recruitment leads to marketing products under the guise of supporting the healthcare industry, providers, and patients. It's an excellent model for creating a massive sustainable, self-growing, and reputable promotion army. What this establishes without a doubt is another element of bias both among healthcare providers as well as public perception complicating true oversight over the SIC.

With the special status of healthcare providers, many skincare products, and brands benefit from the appearance of being healthcare products by proxy, requiring very little to no evidence to support this reputation. According to Wikipedia, an association fallacy is "...an informal inductive fallacy of the hasty-generalization or red-herring type and which asserts, by irrelevant association and often by appeal to emotion, that qualities of one thing are inherently qualities of another. Two types of association fallacies are sometimes guilt by association and honor by association. The SIC's relationship with skincare professionals and academics helps forge an *honor* by association fallacy.

All That Dirt

Most people in the United States, in the Western world, and beyond believe their skin is dirty. In other words, there is a widespread notion skin has dangerous infectious microbes and stuff necessitating cleaning, scrubbing, and anything short of blowtorching it away. How do I know this? The behavior and words of over 99 percent of the tens of thousands of patients I've met over the years.

Do you share this belief? People use a wide array of techniques and products to wage war on this dirt and microbes on their skin. The list includes, but is not limited to, hot water, high pressure shower heads, soap, cleansers, antibacterial compounds, disinfectants, essential oils, scrubs, exfoliants, brushes, sponges, loofah, and more. Physical abrasion, chemical abrasion, disinfection, scalding, and anything in between.

What are we targeting? What is this dirt? The dirt, as we so casually dismiss it, is a highly complex conglomerate, a network of skin resident microbes (bacteria, viruses, fungi, protozoa, mites), human cells (some dead, some in various stages of life), skin-secreted molecules (lipids, proteins, carbohydrates) and some exogenous (outside the body) particles. The function of skin resident dirt is incomprehensible.

This is an unbelievably complex collection of bio-machines, each designed to carry out multiple functions. The term function is often a narrowly applied concept under assuming each cell or even molecule has a singular and well-known role. These so-called machines, for example proteins like filaggrin[31], are versatile and flexible, their downstream effects and interactions complex, no computer can ever reliably simulate their network. I could offer examples of research papers showing microbiome functions, but the findings shown in those articles are a drop in the bucket. While research about the microbiome is important, we must understand its infinitesimal value in making sense of the bigger picture.

This big unknown called the microbiome is an example, an allegory, for our inability to comprehend the impossibly complex and shifting dynamics of biology, our insistence on holding on to some generalization as the ultimate truth. This is human nature, but we can rise above our nature, our impulses, and guesses/answers possibly contrary to our instincts. This brings me to the futility, and danger of putting together synthetic skincare products. We must stop pretending the SIC can simply invent needs SIC-prescribed practices meet. The truth is there's no proven categorical benefit to disrupting, culling, or trimming dirt and the microbiome.

In the past few decades, the SIC has been coming up with more solutions promoted as gentle cleansers. Many of those products use synthetic detergents and other components said or assumed to be less disruptive to skin. As with traditional detergents, there is no significant evidence to support the utility or benefit of gentle cleansers or any cleansers for skin health. Also, one may wonder whether gentle cleansers don't disrupt the upper layers of the skin or not as much as old school detergents, otherwise known as cleaning, what exactly do they do?

In other words, what's the point of gentle cleansing supposedly doing nothing or very little? And if this gentle cleansing does do something, what does it do? The answer: We don't really know. How and why would skincare companies sell and promote products whose benefit and harm are not truly known? The short answer seems complicated. This is a combination of consumer demand, biotechnological advancements, and corporate adaptability. But if I had to boil it down to a bottom-line, making up new problems and creating new solutions is a mechanism for market expansion.

Regardless of the presumed safety of cleansers, I consider them generally a redundant and likely harmful practice. Until proven otherwise, we must view these products with caution. Of particular concern is the wide use of cleansers in children, affecting their skin and likely other aspects of their biology, development, and health.

This brings me to my next point. If there is no dirt on your skin and we are removing a highly complex and little understood element with a blunt hand, what are the consequences? Once again, the answer is: We don't know. Only recently was it conceived that skincare products can induce long-term effects on skin biology, microbiology, possibly other organ biology and function with unknown specifics. This awareness continues to evolve and spread. With all the progress made in uncovering the mystery of skin biology, we are most likely laughably ignorant about the vastly complex effects of skincare products.

However, with recent scientific evidence tying the microbiome to people's skin condition, gut, heart, and even personality we need to tread lightly around skincare, practices, products, and devices. This includes cleansing, cleaning, scrubbing, exfoliation, and other application of chemical or physical manipulation of the skin, hair, and nails. Absence of clear and immediate adversity *does not* equal harmlessness. We simply don't fully understand the big picture consequences of most of what we do to skin. Let's act like it.

Disinfection, Inc.

Here's a radical statement. Your skin is safe. Can you believe it? True, there is a staggering number of microbes living on and in your skin, including fungi, bacteria, viruses, protozoa, mites, and other organisms, overwhelmingly posing no danger to you. They are part of your skin and a part of you. Their well-being is crucial to yours, mostly in ways we don't know or fully understand. The pervasiveness and persistence of the microbiome is a glaring clue to its importance. While we're only beginning to understand the microbiome, I am certain our appreciation and respect for it will grow.

The widespread use of antibacterial compounds and disinfectants, meant to poison and curb the microbiome, is not only unnecessary, but harmful. Disinfection destroys, at least temporarily, and/or alters significant portions of the native microbes, thereby changing their original workings in ways we don't understand. This is troubling since the effects may be as far-reaching as other internal organ systems and the causal connections are challenging to appreciate. Two such systems are the nervous and the reproductive systems, which regulate behavior and our offspring. I believe our individual and even societal skincare habits affect future generations in ways completely incomprehensible to contemporary science. Skincare can influence the microbiome in several ways.

First, skincare alters the function and balance of the existing microbial population, changing the makeup of this element and the interaction with the rest of the skin, the immune system, and the nervous system. These effects stretch across time from the immediate through long term. They ripple, maybe less significantly, from a single use or alternatively form a complex tidal wave with multiple repeated applications of skincare products.

Second, the destruction of parts of the existing microbiome population makes room for other microbial elements to move in, invade the skin, as well as your immediate environment (inanimate objects, pets, other people), and flourish. Nature does not tolerate a vacuum. Something must fill the void the elimination of one element created. Some of those completely new or modified/mutated microbial elements may not have immediate, significant, or noticeable effects. In more extreme circumstances, newly introduced microbes can behave as infectious pathogens, or have other harmful effects such as promotion of irritation, autoimmunity, carcinogenicity, etc.

Third, some antibacterial compounds by themselves have innate toxicity (e.g., triclosan), as well as other properties possibly altering and disrupting normal biology. Those effects may apply to skin, the immune system, the nervous system, or even further anywhere in the body after absorption through the skin, lymph, and capillary systems. Some toxicity is due to effects on the mitochondria, an integral part of most human cells having many similarities to bacteria[32,33,34].

You Work for the SIC and Pay for It

As weird as it may sound at first, the SIC *mostly* gears its biochemical know-how toward serving their products and promoting their own growth over customer needs. Look at the back of most skincare products and you'll find a long list of ingredients, whose names are barely intelligible, much less pronounceable. It takes long months or even years of practice for most dermatologists, let alone laypersons, to wrap their heads around those items. Most of those ingredients, if not all, either preserve the product by maintaining its intended texture/form, inhibiting microbial contamination or enhance the experience of using the product rather than making the product more effective. Manufacturers make products last longer by using preservatives, a structurally diverse category of chemicals maintaining the product in its intended state (molecular chemical structure, texture, smell, color, viscosity, etc.) and prevent microbial growth.

Many different categories of compounds, including but not limited to emulsifiers, stabilizers, fragrances, essential oils, acids, and alcohols to name a few manipulate the product to feel nicer, smell better, or create a specific sensation on the skin. Fulfilling any of these aims *is not* equal to making a better product, e.g., a more effective moisturizer. These intentions are distinct and take away from product efficacy: the product's ability to produce the declared desired effect. This means most ingredients in most commercially available skincare products serve a different purpose or a different master from what the label says. The front label declares servitude of the user's skin. Back labels tell a different story. When most ingredients in a skincare product do not work for the consumer, they serve another master: *The SIC.*

Only a fraction of skincare products is necessary in the first place. Only a fraction of ingredients in those skincare products directly contribute to what the product promises it does, indicating exponentially plummeting value of most skincare products to you. What's even more striking is the premium paid for all those different ingredients incorporated into the skincare products. There are no free lunches. The resources for incorporation of all those ingredients must come from somewhere and rolled over to the consumer.

Examples of such rackets are endless. It's helpful to look at all your products and ask what exactly is their benefit? How do the incorporated ingredients fulfill the product's promise? I invite you to go through this exercise with any one of your skincare products and find out for yourself.

So, when evaluating any skincare product, ask yourself how it truly works for you, whether you even need the declared activity or not. With the ubiquity of products laced with worthless ingredients, regard them with suspicion. Until you have vetted and evaluated the merit of your skincare products, assume the following: The SIC does not work for you. You work for the SIC.

The Fiduciary Relationship of the SIC to its Customers — a Double-edged Sword

Whether you realize it or not, the SIC enjoys the perception of a fiduciary relationship with its customers. Fiduciary relationships form when one party (the fiduciary) acts *on behalf of* another party (the beneficiary) while exercising discretion with respect to a critical resource belonging to the beneficiary. A fiduciary requires all three requirements. Let's examine those criteria with regard to the SIC.

Regarding "on the behalf of" requirement, SIC declaratively manufactures skincare products to benefit the end user, improving or maintaining skin function. According to their own statements, skincare manufacturers are contractors working on behalf of the consumer who buys their products. As a contractor, the manufacturer bundles product development, resource acquisition, production, marketing, sales, and customer service, to name a few elements. This highly complex system's aim is to put the product in the consumers' hands, under the assumption of benefit on their behalf.

What distinguishes a fiduciary is exercising discretion with respect to a critical resource belonging to the beneficiary; most contracting parties exercise discretion only with respect to their own performance under the contract. This is more than just mere access to a resource, differentiating fiduciaries from service providers such as textile manufacturers, receptionists, electricians, and mechanics. The SIC claims to exercise discretion directly by "using the finest ingredients" or implicitly by claiming real or made-up benefits by using a specific product.

The critical resource belonging to the beneficiary is their skin, wellbeing, and beyond, considering the effects of ingredients on skin, skin endocrine secretion, metabolism, the microbiome, and other organ systems.

Another element of the fiduciary relationship of SIC to the customer is the promotion and even sales of skincare products physicians sell to their patients when the fiduciary relationship is traditionally more obvious and the physicians declare themselves as adding a fiduciary-by-proxy factor. So, the SIC has a fiduciary relationship with its customers.

How does the SIC honor this fiduciary responsibility? Let's look at the biggest player as an example. Procter & Gamble[35] states the following: "Safety is at the heart of everything we do. Before we market a new product, we go beyond regulatory compliance to ensure every ingredient's safety through a four-step, science-based process. We use the same process as regulatory agencies around the world, like the U.S. FDA, EPA, the EU, the WHO, and others." They outline their product safety assurance process in four steps.

Step one: "Doubt" involves P&G scientists raising questions regarding ingredient benefit and safety. In theory, this is a good idea. The problem is we can only study what we are aware of and have the resources to engage.

Step two: "Define" is detailing an "ingredient's safe range using the same science-based standards as major regulatory agencies around the world."

Step three: "Determine." They "evaluate all ingredients in the product to ensure they are safe when used both for you and the environment. If we can't confirm that, we go back to the drawing board." This is obviously an impossible task to achieve. The concept of safety changes with our understanding of biology. Testing environmental impact is also impossible as it is too complex a question to answer.

Step four: "Diligence" is the most honest step acknowledged on P&G's list and involves keeping up with new findings regarding their ingredients, which they acknowledge is "never-ending." This is correct and points to the bigger picture regarding the fluid definition of safety and benefit.

Declaratively, the SIC engages in practices designed to ensure product safety and benefit down to the ingredients. But is this really the case? While it's impossible to make any generalizations, we can investigate specific cases. Let's look at examples of Regenerist Day Face Cream, a popular product by

Olay™, a subsidiary of P&G Co.[36] containing 50 listed ingredients. In the U.S., a similar product called Regenerist Micro-Sculpting Cream Moisturizer[37] contains 28 listed ingredients.

Let's examine the integrity of the fiduciary relationship, and how corporate holds its end of the bargain. In other words, we'll see whether the attitudes of the SIC toward product claims, ingredient benefit, and safety hold water.

These are the promises Olay makes regarding Regenerist Day Face Cream.

Look at these claims and carefully crafted messages and examine for logical and factual accuracy.

<u>Statement</u>: *"Daily face cream visibly renews your skin's natural glow."*

<u>Factually</u>: The human skin doesn't have a natural glow. In fact, glowing human skin is decidedly abnormal and is either achieved artificially or in certain pathologies, such as hyperhidrosis (excessive sweating) or excessive oil production, which is often a reaction to skincare abuse.

<u>Statement</u>: *"Fine, velvety texture, ideal for dry to combination skin."*

<u>Factually</u>: Function, not texture, makes any product or application a fit for a skin type. Which brings us to the next point: Dry skin requires emollience, occlusion, and, at times, a humectant for the best moisturizing results, making this product not ideal as we will see below. Second, combination skin is almost always the result of chronic skincare abuse with misdirected grooming, such as cleansing, scrubbing, and more. This is one example of the SIC creating a problem with one set of products and coming to the rescue with another: a fireman's arson.

<u>Statement</u>: *"Formulated with Vitamin B3 & amino peptides, two powerful skincare ingredients."*

Factually: First, there is no such thing as amino peptides[38]. All peptides are made up of amino acids, so the word amino is redundant, either erroneously added or inserted for promotional considerations, sprinkling more pseudo-science into the language. Data supporting the topical application and utility of vitamin B3 and peptides[39] appears in a few low-level publications. This means the statement "powerful skincare ingredients" is unsubstantiated and requires more evidence. Also, what undesired, unintended effects can these two powerful ingredients have? We don't know.

Statement: *"Delivers active ingredients 10 layers deep into skin surface."*

Factually: This claim needs specification and backing. What 10 layers and how do the products traverse them? The epidermis and dermis amount to a total of seven layers. What is the drawback of increased permeability of their product? What active ingredients? Yes, there are two ingredients mentioned by name, but those are not separate as active ingredients so no one can know what the active ingredients in this product are and what their function is. Also, the systemic absorption and effects of those active and inactive ingredients are unclear.

Statement: *"Intensely hydrates skin for 24 hours."*

Factually: What does "intensely hydrates" mean? And how is the 24-hour effect assessed? Interestingly, even occlusive stable moisturizers such as petrolatum require more than one daily application in many cases.

Statement: *"Improves skin texture by encouraging surface cell renewal."*

Factually: Encouraging surface cell renewal is a nebulous term. More pseudo-science sprinkled in. What surface cells are we discussing, and just as importantly which ones are we not? How is renewal defined and measured? How does the effect relate to skin texture? If it does, is it the most significant factor affecting skin texture in this product?

Statement: *"Use daily for 28 days. See true skin appearance transformation."*

Factually: How did they arrive at this "28 days" magical number? What is the specific transformation in skin appearance?

Regenerist Works for Olay — Judge Them by Their Actions Not Their Words

As we'll clarify in the following discussion, most ingredients in Regenerist, if not all (as well as countless other products) are to support manufacturer needs, rather than the customer's needs. If you scroll through the list of ingredients once again, you will mostly see a plethora of items whose function is to stabilize the product, preserve, or shape the product experience, whether it's color/sparkle, scent, or texture. The ingredients claimed to benefit skin are in unknown quantities, and their skin benefits are unclear, especially in topical form. All this begs the question for whom do the ingredients truly work? Unless there is a proven and clear skin benefit to an ingredient, it works for the manufacturer at the customer's expense, literally.

Regenerist Day Face Cream has no less than fifty ingredients. According to P&G's four D's one may presume the company thoroughly vetted those chemicals for safety, as well as benefit to the customer.

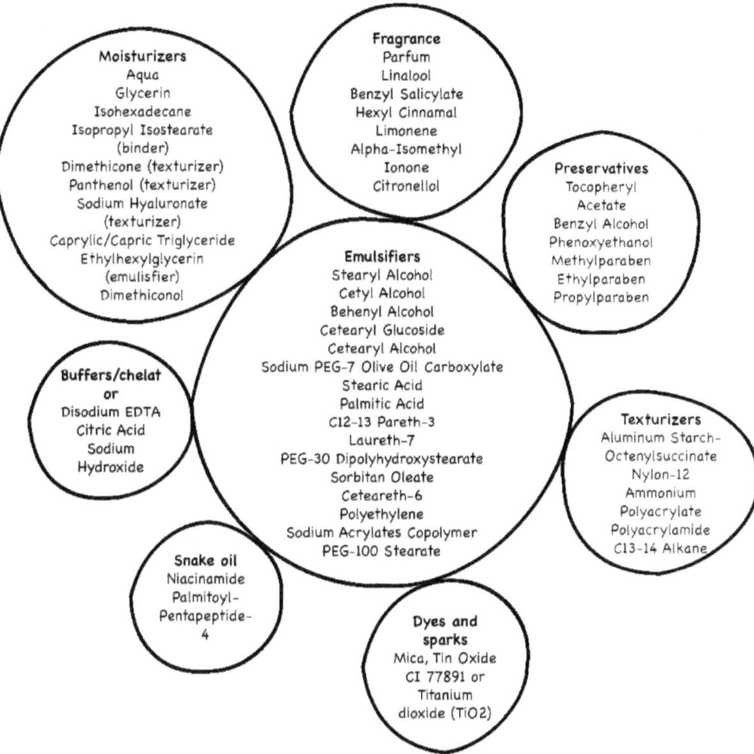

Figure 1. Regenerist Day Face Cream ingredient list by category. Some ingredients may serve several functions as indicated in parenthesis[40,41].

Examining the figure above is an eye-opening experience. Notice how most ingredients serve roles other than moisturization (not the claimed function of the product) or snake oils, which are the formula's claim to fame. With no less than fifteen emulsifiers (there are more considering multifunctional ingredients), seven fragrance additives (some of which are likely composed of more than one molecule), six preservatives (!), and two compounds adding to visual appearance, it's shocking to see how much of this product does not serve its declared purpose.

Take the time to review this ingredient list and ask yourself once again, for whom does this product work? Who is paying? Remember, you work for the SIC and pay for it.

The Scam of Active vs. Inactive Ingredients

Active ingredients in skincare products must confer some benefit to the user, even when they have clear associated side effects, e.g., the compound adapalene. Adapalene is a retinoid, now available over the counter in the United States. This medication and other medications in its class, mainly used to treat acne, can cause dryness and irritation of the treated skin. This is an obvious relationship between a clearly beneficial ingredient and direct side effects of its use.

With so-called inactive ingredients, the relationship becomes messy. "Inactive ingredient" is a misnomer, a fallacy because there would be no reason to invest resources and use an ingredient that is inactive or serves no function. There is no such thing as an inactive ingredient since any chemical has an activity, though sometimes challenging to assess and determine. In the case of the SIC, rest assured incorporating every so-called inactive ingredient is cost-effective. The function of inactive ingredients is to serve the manufacturer at the user's expense. Preservatives, emulsifiers, texturizers, dyes, fragrance, and snake oil serve a technical or a promotional function that does not add benefit to the product. Preservatives may add a level of safety when there is a concern for contamination of the product by dangerous pathogens, which is rare. One can claim an emulsifier is important in maintaining the activity of a product. However, emulsifiers/surfactants can disrupt cell membranes, extracellular oils, and increase skin permeability, leading to altered skin function as well as loss of moisture.

Our understanding of the gamut of side effects of inactive ingredients is rife with blind spots: the unexplored — what we know we don't know and unimagined — what we don't know we don't know. This unwilful and willful ignorance undermines the fiduciary relationship between SIC and its customers: adding unbeneficial ingredients to skincare products with unsuspecting customers fully paying for them.

Most skincare products, especially those promoted by arbitrary recommendations, violate the fiduciary relationship. There are varying degrees of violation, depending on what the company declares the product can do (as opposed to what it actually does), as well as the net active ingredient composition of the product as opposed to inactive ingredients and their effect on the skin and beyond. As D. Gordon Smith[42] puts it as the beginning of his essay: "...fiduciary law is messy." Certainly, fiduciary relationships, whether legally binding or not, are complex and can be ambiguous. The SIC shares a fiduciary association with its customers and paradoxically violates it with various SIC strategies. Those include making false or exaggerated claims and a compulsion to incorporate self-serving inactive ingredients into products at the customer's expense.

Many inactive ingredients make the product more appealing, which is a legitimate goal. People buy products they like using. What is not legitimate is undermining the declared purpose of the product. Understandably, the SIC spends its public relations resources blurring and disguising this point. Being upfront about this would be akin to putting the less than savory truth in the spotlight.

But why would making a product more appealing affect its efficacy? Let's do the math. The product's efficacy is measurable by the proportion of influence of active ingredients, fulfilling the main goal of the product to the influence of inactive ingredients, fulfilling aims other than the product's goal. The more influence inactive ingredients exert, the less effective a product is. This is a reductive distillation of composition efficacy. When we get down to particulars, it's much trickier to determine the weight of inactive ingredients on efficacy.

Not all inactive ingredients are equal. Some may simply take up volume not directly and actively affecting the function of the active ingredients or the skin's integrity. Other ingredients may have a negative impact either directly on the function of active ingredients or indirectly by damaging skin integrity.

The significance of such effects not only ties to volume but also to chemical properties of such inactive ingredients. Beyond diluting the declared product function, inactive ingredients can lead to irritation, toxicity, and microbiome interference, as examples.

Let's take moisturizers, for example. Making a greasy moisturizer creamier decreases its efficacy, possibly even increases TEWL. Ingredients solely incorporated to make a moisturizer smell a certain way add no moisturizing value and potentially make the product less safe. Preservatives, which are extremely common additives, do not increase efficacy either and may have many adverse effects.

Aquaphor Healing Ointment — "Product Appeal" Dilutes Value

Take, for example, Aquaphor Healing Ointment (AHO[43]), considered an excellent moisturizer by many dermatologists. AHO is relatively greasy, which is what gives long-lasting moisturization. On the other hand, AHO is not too greasy, making it more enjoyable to use than petroleum jelly for many. More enjoyable or appealing does not equal more effective, chipping away at efficacy. AHO has a very delicate medicinal odor, and its shelf life is virtually indefinite. Let's look at the ingredient list.

The only active ingredient is *petrolatum* (petroleum jelly), making up 41 percent of the product. Petrolatum is an excellent occlusive moisturizer, effective, safe, cheap. On the inactive ingredient list is mineral oil, ceresin, lanolin alcohol, panthenol, glycerin, and bisabolol. The company likely incorporated the first five ingredients on the inactive list to create the "right texture." This comes at the expense of petrolatum, cutting into its occlusive effect. Those still have value as moisturizing elements, just not as effective as petrolatum. So, in this case a more "appealing" texture equals a less effective product. Most egregious is bisabolol, a fragrance compound, with no skin moisturizing value, which could be a potential allergen.

AHO is an example of one of the better ratios of active to inactive ingredients. Most skincare products contain an overwhelming majority of ingredients exclusively serving the manufacturer's needs.

More startling examples of so-called inactive ingredients are in products whose claim to fame are the very ingredients listed as inactive. Two examples are Regenerist Whip Face Moisturizer by Olay[44] and CeraVe Healing Ointment[45]. On its website right above the ingredient list, the following statement says: "Our favorite ingredient at Olay is Vitamin B3. This ingredient is known to help skin retain moisture keeping it seriously hydrated. Vitamin B3 can also hydrate to help with surface skin cell turnover and regeneration, as well as exfoliation to remove dull skin. Long story short — it's our unicorn."

Right below is the following claim: "Amino peptides are chains of amino acids and the building blocks of skin cells. These boss babe molecules are known to help skin look smoother and firmer." However, the product ingredient list, just a few lines below, lists Niacinamide and Vitamin B3 (synonymous) as well as palmitoyl pentapeptide-4 and peptide as inactive ingredients. So, the "boss babe molecules" and the "unicorn" are not up to much when it comes to the consumer.

CeraVe pulls a similar trick with its healing ointment. Listing ceramides right under the "Skin Protectant" claim on the product package creating an association between the two, as well as stating their product is "lightweight yet intensely hydrating and features three essential ceramides and hyaluronic acid in a moisturizing base." However, the product ingredient list tells a different story with ceramide np, ceramide ap, ceramide eop, as well as hyaluronic acid all listed as "Inactive Ingredients."

The Meaning of "Science" in SIC-Speak

Abandoning categorical and automated skincare practices takes a leap of faith. This is more than a figure of speech. Many people practice skincare as religious rites or rituals. This is the religion of perfect skin.

Every religious narrative seeking to sustain, fortify, and propagate itself, uses language to do so. Let's look at the SIC use of language to manipulate the meaning of words and promote its products. It's what I've come to call SIC-speak. One consistently harnessed term is "science," or rather the mention of science and things pertaining to it. While scientific discovery certainly drives innovation, including skincare, we must distinguish between the true concept of science and the science or scientific and pseudoscientific terms used in SIC propaganda and marketing. With the glorification of science, the mention of the term gives a product or a practical concept an air of respectability.

According to Wikipedia, science is "is a systematic enterprise that builds and organizes knowledge in the form of testable explanations and predictions about the universe"[46]. Science is a specific term, and the scientific method is uncompromising. Unfortunately, over the past few decades, there has been a significant loosening in the use of the word to various ends. People who do this understand science, choosing to manipulate its meaning, as well as people who do not understand the term or its underlying principles, throwing it around cavalierly just the same.

Science is a wonderful tool for discovery. It also has limits for a variety of reasons, having to do with the physics of space, time, and energy, combined with the staggering complexity of nature. This is *not* a dismissal of science but rather a warning regarding common abuse of the term. Here are some examples of the inherent limitations of science.

First, scientific studies can only focus on one or a limited number of testable questions or hypotheses. Usually, the researcher's interest and available resources restrict them. Second, the investigated models limit research, whether it's a cell culture, an animal model, people, or a computer simulation, for example. Third, most scientific observations have limited application to the vast, infinite, and ever-shifting biological diversity as well as the people interpreting the findings, implementing their own skincare approach. Fourth, not all scientific findings are equal. Some studies are well designed, and executed, while some are not, with most falling somewhere in the middle.

So, not all data are equally valid or valuable. Even extraordinary studies have a way of getting it wrong or falsification. There is a fully blown problem in the scientific world, known as the reproducibility crisis[47] where others cannot replicate many studies. This goes almost completely unnoticed, but it has serious consequences in the real world, including skincare.

Fifth, because of the complexity of biology, scientific conclusion (and common perception) must deal in averages, generalities, and approximation, while life is particular. Every case is unique, even when very similar to other cases. So, the best science can do is provide an estimation of how things play out, which is often a mistake for prediction and certainty.

In many ways, this is very useful. Getting a general sense of biology helps understand disease and develop solutions for very common categories of conditions. But efficacy differs from case to case, from treatment period to treatment period. As any experienced physician will tell you, there are numerous people whose "very common" conditions do not respond to conventional treatments with great track records. There are no perfect "one size fits all" solutions for most medical problems. This applies across *all* categories of medicine. For example, minocycline, an antibiotic which works in many cases of inflammatory acne, may achieve complete clearance in one patient and only a moderate improvement in another. Also, a patient achieving complete clearance may experience occasional flareups or become resistant to treatment.

Sixth, scientists, policy makers, corporate executives, and laypeople cherry pick so-called scientific evidence and derived conclusions to support their agenda or due to other biases. Ideally, the scientific method is meant to eliminate bias. In the real world, the word science can mean many things, often curated statements in support of an agenda under the guise of irrefutable truth.

If you revisit much of the promotional material the SIC uses over the past few decades, you'll notice there are plenty of references to science, scientific breakthroughs, precision, and "secrets." There are colorful graphics and special effects creating an image of cutting-edge technology making your skin a utopian better place. Celebrities, often altered surgically, cosmetically, and digitally, promote insider skincare tips, mysterious doctors tout miraculous discoveries of natural fountain of youth molecules found in melons. Most of those claims have no scientific backing, or in other words, they are *hogwash*.

How much "science" truly goes into skincare product design? The science driving skincare production is the science of marketing, consisting of a variety of flavors of psychology, geared toward persuasion and conversion. Much of this mechanism is geared towards finding or manufacturing consumption gaps to fill, promptly providing solutions, as in the example of the Pepsodent Effect[48], which I'll discuss shortly. A product designed to sell well is not necessarily effective — or even safe. Many ingredients used in skincare products have a dubious track record[49], as most skincare products have questionable benefits. So, when SIC uses the term science or terms sounding scientific it does not mean science. The closest approximation of what this verbal handwaving means is "buy our product or you're going to miss out on the newest, shiniest technology for your skin." This paints a product in a reliable, safe, and beneficial light. A splash of urgency creates FOMO. It is nothing more than a persuasion tool. So, if science doesn't quite mean what you think it means in SIC-speak, what does safe mean? Let's break it down.

The Meaning of "Safe" in SIC-Speak

The public considers skincare products safe with a pervasive belief that skincare products won't have adverse consequences. Otherwise, we wouldn't use them. It seems most people do not consider their skincare products to possess any risk whatsoever. But how do you really know the product you're using is safe? And what does safe really mean? Literally nothing is without risk. Everything you do (or don't do) and every product you use, has some risk of adverse effects, even if negligible or immeasurable at present. The goalposts of what is safe are an ever-shifting standard. This safety index depends on many factors, including the available data, as well as public perception. When new information presents itself or public opinion shifts, so do safety standards.

So, what does safe mean in SIC-speak? What do skincare manufacturers truly mean when they claim their products are safe? In SIC-speak, the word safe means per the interpretation of our measurements we can live with the potential side effect profile. So, safety is a limited liability term. Personally, I am not terribly worried about this. If we know what the term means, anyone can use a product at their own risk. But what about the benefit of skincare? Let's examine the cleansing category.

Couldn't Hurt

One of the leading conscious and unconscious assumptions almost every person using skincare products makes is product harmlessness. What's the origin of the belief? First, the SIC has a fiduciary relationship with customers, implicitly at least. This infuses the SIC/customer relationship with fundamental and pervasive sense of trust among customers to use products with blind faith in their benefit and harmlessness.

Second, in most cases, commercial skincare products are *visibly* well-tolerated immediately and even long-term, meaning the product does not produce a sustained irritant reaction, the most common measure, e.g., burning, itchiness, redness, swelling, and flakiness.

Third, especially in the Western world, people assume manufacturers test, vet, and certify skincare products safe and regulatory government agencies guarantee safety. This is a largely implicit assumption rooted in the fiduciary relationship. However, testing standards vary by product, company, country, and time period, which translates into the technology used, scope of investigation/testing, and conclusions based on contemporary knowledge and social trends.

The breadth of testing is a gray area. "Thoroughly tested" is a dynamic and variable term. Moreover, government regulation of skincare is rife with issues making it a largely illusory concept, including the innate ineffective nature of government and lack of linear moral accountability in government bureaucracies. The FDA website states: "FDA does not have the legal authority to approve cosmetic products and ingredients (other than color additives) before they go on the market. We also do not have a list of tests required for any cosmetic product or ingredient."[50]

What are all those products tested for and how? It's difficult to evaluate exactly what skincare companies do to test their products, for several reasons:

- Product testing is an extremely complex and truly a never-ending process (as honestly acknowledged by P&G, for example). This can include review of previous scientific evidence of ingredient safety, actual testing by the manufacturer through in-vitro, animal, or human experiments and finally, ongoing review of ingredient and product safety post-marketing. This means product testing stretches into infinity as we learn new data, products, ingredients, and our scientific methods improve. Testing is just testing — a sampling of an ongoing process giving a snapshot idea of the state of things. It is not a failsafe mechanism; things can go wrong before or after quality and safety testing of a product.

- Product testing is not transparent. This is due to multiple factors, including trade secrets and proprietary knowledge, little political/ public interest manifesting as very lax enforcement of standards, corporate interest in containing/cleaning the image of a very intricate and easily misinterpreted process, as well as corporate ever-shifting focus on issues other than consumer safety. Such issues include political and social activism.[51] The ever-growing focus of corporate executives on activism is killing two birds with one stone: gaining some public favor and effectively shifting attention from potentially worrisome issues such as product safety, as well as the environmental impact of the industry.[52]

- Safety testing on its many forms is shortsighted and narrow in scope, mostly focusing on immediate effects of products locally at the application site. There is very little consideration given to systemic effects and long-term effects because studying them would be exorbitantly costly, lengthy, or beyond the test's scope. You simply cannot test for "everything" or know the future ramifications of years or decades of use for everyone.

- Our understanding of what is "safe" keeps evolving, as it should. Factors like the microbiome, for example, were not and are likely still not a prominent consideration in development and deployment of skincare products and their respective ingredients. As our understanding of the importance of the microbiome grows,[53] as well as other unknown and undiscovered factors become known, it's clear the scientific and medical communities don't fully grasp the ramifications of using skincare products.

Regarding the microbiome, I question the harmlessness of the widespread use of preservatives and antibacterial ingredients in skincare. Beyond designated preservatives and antimicrobials, we have a poor understanding of other ingredients, such as emulsifiers, surfactants, dyes, fragrances, and other compound categories on the microbiome and its relationship to skin, as well as skin metabolites. This is an endless question since each individual compound or chemical has a unique interaction with different people's microbiome, likely specific to distinct body regions on the same person.

Our understanding of biology has limits and continues to evolve. The collected knowledge is growing much more slowly and with limits than we give science and technology credit. Scientific inquiry continues. But above all, it is important to cultivate a sense of humility in our ability to truly evaluate the effects of anything we do or experience on biology, more specifically human health, an infinitely chaotically complex and ever-shifting concept. The skincare industry must approach its development and manufacturing process with a greater sense of humility and sanctity.

Whatever your belief system, you must acknowledge the ungraspable complexity of biology and the human body. Trillions of human cells working with tenfold more numerous microbes to create a perfect, sustainable harmony. The sophistication of this biological orchestra, the human being, is a marvel (whatever narrative you choose to believe). Skincare products are factory produced. They should show much more reverence for the body.

But let's not kid ourselves. The SIC will not change direction any time soon. In fact, the SIC is more likely to double down on snake oil, irresponsible production, and marketing, as well as virtue signaling to distract from their sins. It is up to us, the intended recipients of SIC propaganda and end users of their products to wise up. We must use our judgment and determine what is truly beneficial for our skin.

The Meaning of Natural in SIC-Speak

In everyday discourse, the word natural is now associated with or even equal to essential, beneficial, safe, or harmless. This is a fallacy, conflating natural with good. A snide joke among dermatologists about the natural and organic product market is poison ivy is natural, non-GMO, and organic. Condescending humor aside, not everything found in nature, even molecules or compounds occurring in your own body, or even in the skin itself are necessarily advantageous when topically applied. Why?

Nature and specifically biology are systems of balance and boundaries between different elements, water, ions, proteins, carbohydrates, lipids, and others. There is a time, form, quantity, and place for everything. Biological systems, skin included, evolved to take and use what they need to function and carry out their purpose: keeping things they don't need away or inactivating them.

Another fact you already know intuitively is most natural ingredients do not occur in nature. Most natural products are mass-produced, heavily processed, refined concoctions of ingredients, many of which companies throw together for promotional and industrial reasons, e.g., marketing and preservation. Essential oils aren't natural. They are highly complex mixtures of distilled plant concentrates. Commercially available vitamins are either synthetically produced or heavily processed from natural resources. Even plant-based oils or butters are physically and often chemically extracted and purified. There are varying degrees of processing, many of which change the original natural chemical composition of those compounds and mixtures. So, natural isn't truly natural, but rather pretending to be natural with the occasional origin in a natural resource.

Assuming any one ingredient or an ingredient category can repair sensitive or damaged skin, or that it is in exactly the needed form and quantities in a mass-produced moisturizer, is naïve at best. But the SIC relies exactly on the general public assumption and even skincare professionals to promote many of their products as beneficial. In most cases, this is no more than a marketing ploy.

Skincare Strikes a Primal Chord

Looking good and feeling good about one's image is a basic human need. Most people make a decent effort to look attractive, whether it's for work, friends, romance, or fitting in generally. This human impulse is recession proof, as economic downturns appear to increase women's spending on beauty products, a phenomenon termed the lipstick effect.[54] Motivations driving skincare are complex and powerful, from apparently inherent personal impulses through societal cues, pressures, and fashion trends.

Skincare promotion is fertile ground for breeding habits, rooted in generic often baseless assertions, frequently forming obsessive-compulsive vicious cycles. Meaning, a person could be repeatedly and stubbornly applying skincare in a harmful manner, strongly believing this is addressing the very problem that the practice reinforces or even creates. Take, for example, the ritual of scrubbing, which physically traumatizes the skin, expecting the skin to "rejuvenate."

In my own life, I was in no way free from those assumptions and resulting practices. Like most of the people I now counsel, I fell for many SIC propaganda tropes. For many years, I shampooed my hair most days with or without conditioning, clueless about the effects of each product, believing it was "good for me." I soaped from face to toe every time I showered, as well as used cleansers, scrubs, exfoliants, and even a brush on my face. I would walk by a sink and feel compelled to wash my hands just for the heck of it. None of those practices made things better. Many of them made my skin worse, which didn't stop me from carrying on for years or even decades. I did this mostly without much thought, all the while believing on some level those practices were good for me.

In my internship hospital, the administration encouraged frequent washing or disinfection of the hands with the slogan "FOAM BEFORE YOU ROAM," printed on signs hung over alcohol foam dispensers which were everywhere. I followed this direction, wanting to be a team player. Every time I passed a dispenser, I pushed the nob to release a silver-dollar sized amount of foam, rubbed it on my hands and let it dry. After a couple of weeks of foaming and roaming, I developed ichthyosis of the hands, with the skin turning into fishlike scale. My skin was so dry, cracked, and sensitive, I had to almost stop any washing, cleansing, or foaming completely inside and outside the hospital. It was simply too painful. I ended up using disposable gloves, applying disinfectant to the gloves. The painful cracks and fishlike skin went away within a couple of weeks, and I learned a valuable lesson regarding reflexive skincare. Do everything intentionally, moderately, and the cure cannot be worse than the disease.

The Hook — The Foundations of Forming an Addiction to Skincare

Tony Robbins defined six human needs as: certainty, uncertainty (or variety), love and connection, significance, growth, and contribution.[55] According to Robbins, anything meeting at least three of those needs may become an addiction. When examining the business model of the SIC, subscribing to the contemporary skincare prescriptive package appears to meet those needs, including the promise of perfect (or better) skin and its broader association with a better multifaceted life.

SIC propaganda targets several of those needs, including certainty, significance, growth, connection. SIC propaganda includes even uncertainty in the form of variety, pleasant surprises, or serendipity. The promise for perfect skin by the SIC has created a whole universe of superstition, masquerading as a factual cause and effect narrative, as seen in countless personal beauty blogs and SIC websites. Bloggers, advertisers, skincare professionals, acquaintances, and naturally, skincare companies tout the health benefits of countless ingredients, products, and techniques with the utmost authority. This authority, or confidence, infuses a sense of certainty in target audiences, as well as create the impression of growth in understanding of their own skin and the skin of others. This movement has spawned a booming skin expert industry. This is largely a make-believe world. The so-called experts are mostly promoters of dubious skincare habits, rather than true authorities. Just the same, SIC promotion is virtually inescapable and seductive.

The SIC uses the experience of using skincare products to create another layer of certainty, through beautiful packaging, specific colors and fragrance, and sensations those products induce. The scent of many skincare products, most of which are not perfumes or deodorants, trains customers in identifying correct or desirable smells. The SIC created or at least amplified the significance of standards for correct skin texture or tone. Countless users of skincare products strive toward perfectly smooth skin, which is unrealistic and undesirable. The SIC determined this standard but made it look as if it were your idea. Cultivating a sense of what's the correct skin feeling, such as fresh (irritated skin) is another category of manipulation the SIC employs.

Those standards are by design promoting certainty about how your skin should be, look, and feel. Flowing from certainty, the experience of using skincare products can then answer other requirements. Using skincare products for grooming, can enhance significance (getting attention and compliments), uncertainty (increase the variety of people one's likely to meet), connection (meet like-minded people, business, or romantic prospects), and growth (making oneself and others better). It is also a source of connection by sharing beauty tips, exchanging compliments, or enhancing attractiveness.

Especially in the past two or three decades, the SIC's seizure of social justice has given consumers the impression they are part of a movement for a better world. Buy a tube of lotion and save the rain forest. Shave your face and fight toxic masculinity. Recyclable materials, natural ingredients, organic, non-GMO, fair trade, leading to an inflation of virtue signaling. This targets the need for significance, certainty, contribution, and connection.

Many skincare routines, systems, or recommendations have a cult-like following with customers becoming a major part of their promotion effort, converting other people to buying in. Significance, certainty, contribution, connection, growth. Great examples are the Proactiv system (potentially using celebrity endorsements to develop a cult-like sense of belonging, etc.), as well as various makeup lines, e.g., CoverGirl, Mac, and Maybelline.

Many have experienced the insistence of a family member or a friend about a new must have, "life changing" skincare system. Whether it was through bragging about their own improvement, the promise of sustaining great skin, slowing, or stopping aging, this is a widespread phenomenon. The reverse can also occur, for example, a friend envious of your perfect skin soliciting beauty tips.

Up until recently, this was decidedly in the domain of womanhood. However, over the past two decades, this trend has increasingly encroached on the lives and conversations of men, pushing the SIC into new frontiers.

Another consequence of sweeping statements is relinquishment of individual agency and the freedom to choose. However, one-size-fits-all is a myth. And while there's nothing wrong with making a profit, there are additional factors weighing in, including the product or service sold and claims made about it. Capitalism and sustainable free markets require virtue and morals to offset unchecked greed and other human vices. This is true for both business and consumers. The SIC has abdicated virtue as well as morals and replaced them with virtue signaling. These are mutually exclusive. Focusing on actual virtues like charity and humility stands in contrast to virtue signaling, which is the embodiment of vices such as pride, greed, and envy. It's either one or the other. Regrettably, the SIC has largely chosen narcissism over doing the right thing.

The SIC-Pepsodent Effect — the Experience-Based Skincare Promotion Leading to Habit Formation

Many skincare products, such as abrasives, (for example: Old Spice Men's Body Wash Deep Cleanse with Deep Sea Minerals and Aveeno Positively Radiant Skin Brightening Exfoliating Daily Facial Scrub) immediately undermine skin integrity, prompting sensations such as tightness, burning, itch, as well as causing redness or even "glow." The SIC has worked hard to link those sensations with buzzwords such as brightening, radiant, fresh or awake, implicitly beneficial.

In many cases, this is a marketing strategy, like the Pepsodent toothpaste campaign. In the early 1900s, Claude Hopkins, a marketing executive created a brilliant strategy to promote Pepsodent toothpaste. Reading through dentistry textbooks, Hopkins found his cue in the form of mucinous plaque coating teeth. He called the phenomenon "film," problematized it, dubbing it "a dangerous coating that robs teeth of their whiteness" and offered a solution (despite no evidence of utility) in the toothpaste he promoted.

Pepsodent had another ace up its sleeve, adding mint oil and citric acid to their tooth cleaning products, creating a tingly feeling inside the mouth. While having no health benefit, this sensation made customers feel good about brushing their teeth, leading to an explosion in Pepsodent product sales, transforming the oral care industry forever. Within a decade of the campaign launch, Pepsodent toothpaste among Americans went from 7 percent to over 65 percent. This scheme had several notable elements.[56]

First, it focused on a natural widespread phenomenon and created a need to fix it by problematizing it, i.e., "the dangerous film making teeth yellow." Second, it offered a solution and attached an immediate "reward" to its use, toothpaste infused with irritants creating a physical sensation, reinforcing perceived product value. The physical effect needn't have any direct benefit, as in the case of Pepsodent.

Many skincare products use a similar marketing strategy designed to create an experience-based narrative. The most common problematization of naturally occurring skin phenomena is dubbing the upper layers of the skin as dirt or oil. Products such as soaps, cleansers, scrubs, exfoliants, masks, brushes, or rollers induce irritation physically and/or chemically by disrupting the skin's upper layers. The effect in many cases feels like "tightening" of the skin, which has become synonymous with buzzwords or phrases such as fresh and "wake up call." Like the Pepsodent effect, the resulting sensation serves to reinforce the regular use of the product, thereby forming a habit. Consequently, the SIC uses the fresh and cleansing effects much like the toothpaste industry used the Pepsodent effect. Unlike the toothpaste and oral care industry, the benefit of cleansing and refreshing skincare products is dubious.

Chapter 4:
A Look at Cleansing

The 19th and 20th centuries exploded with many scientific discoveries in a wide range of fields, including physics, chemistry, biology, and hybrid fields such as biotechnology, high-tech, and so on. Many of those breakthroughs transformed society and the way people live. Establishing the relationship between microbes and infection, along with antimicrobial pharmaceutical and biochemical advancements helped save *millions of lives* by *preventing* and *curing* infection.

Two major industries that benefitted were food and healthcare, both plagued with microbial pathology acting as a largely untamed force of nature causing significant morbidity and death. Indeed, those industries had great incentives to implement all sorts of antimicrobial measures.

When I was in medical school, we discussed microbes mainly in the context of infectious disease prevention and treatment. There was little mention of "good bacteria" and the concept of the microbiome was barely known, let alone mentioned. Except for the development of antibiotic resistance, no one even considered other possible downsides to disinfection, sterilization, or antibiotic use.

Things began to take a turn for the worse when the attitudes prevailing in the healthcare and food industry seeped into society at large. This attitude has dominated Western culture and beyond for decades, leading to the explosion in healthy household use of antibacterial soaps, disinfectants, and antibiotics.[57] Many in Western countries mindlessly employ all those technologies to prevent infection, while completely oblivious to any possible disadvantages in this approach.

In healthcare, the prevailing sentiment curbing indiscriminate use of antibiotics was fear of emerging bacterial resistance. Otherwise, most people, including physicians, were more than happy to disinfect and sanitize their way through life, including family members and children. Social media with its wide-open platforms and ease of idea dissemination seems to play a large role in the spread of those attitudes, completely transforming the culture. Handwashing with antibacterial soap, surface wipe-downs, and use of over-the-counter antimicrobials are now an automatic norm for countless people.

To date, the only major speed bumps to this trend are discoveries regarding harmful effects of certain antibacterials on human health and the environment. One example is triclosan. Triclosan has been in use since the 1970s, but reports regarding its hormonal effects, allergenic potential, or environmental burden began emerging in the late 1990s and early 2000s. Government agencies finally acted *more than a decade later*, with the FDA banning the use of triclosan among other compounds in over-the-counter antiseptic wash products in 2016.[58] Following this decision, companies quietly phased out products containing triclosan and replaced it with other antibacterial compounds such as benzalkonium chloride (Trade name Zephiran).

Triclosan is an example of human ingenuity, misused due to greed, arrogance, and pride. It is by no means an isolated case. As we learn more about the less obvious effects of various traditional skincare ingredients, public awareness increases, and more ingredients will phase out. This does not mean an end to disinfection, but simply shifting of technology, complying with regulatory guidelines, as well as public perceptions.

The triclosan debacle is a drop in the bucket of the harm caused by the handwashing and disinfection craze. The obsession with cleanliness has bred a pandemic of sensitive, dry skin, as well as atopy: a tendency to develop various allergic and reactive conditions, such as asthma, and eczema. Further downstream consequences, such as effects on endocrine health, cardiovascular health, and mental health are virtually unknown. Yet the antibacterial craze has only worsened with more products and more frequent application use, with the COVID 19-pandemic "disinfection boom" sprouting on fertile ground, primed for decades, almost unabated. The pandemic reset the baseline to a far more involved culture of cleaning rituals.

Now, the SIC is certainly aware of at least some of the adverse effects of its products, namely dryness and irritation induced or worsened by detergents and abrasives used in cleansing. So how did the SIC deal with this realization of harm a wide range of its products causes? Let's examine how the SIC can have its cake and eat it too through a combination of technological innovation and clever word games.

Cleansing as a Redundant Misnomer

I frequently hear from patients that they thoroughly clean themselves from head to toe, using a shampoo/conditioner combination for the scalp, a gentle cleanser (a made-up concept minted to reassure people and increase use) for the face, a body wash, or a soap for the rest, as well as all sorts of abrasive, physical scrubbing devices. And let's not forget hot water. As you'll recall, I was a devout follower of this approach for many years.

There is literally no evidence of a health benefit to the thorough cleaning, cleansing, and other head to toe grooming rituals most of society advocates and practices, including many skincare professionals. So, head to toe cleansing is unnecessary and potentially harmful. Now, I'd like to focus on the cleansing practice with a positive impact on human health — handwashing.

First, the facts. Handwashing, with or without soap, *decreases* microbial counts generally and can decrease transmission of infectious disease when pathogens are on the skin. So, handwashing makes sense when dealing with a dangerous infectious pathogen, especially in communities ravaged by contagious gastrointestinal and skin illness, as well as industries like food and healthcare. While it's not a foolproof tool to prevent transmission of infection with variations in efficacy of handwashing, it is important in several settings. However, there are caveats to handwashing and cleaning that require a discerning approach. With every beneficial measure, there are also undesired and unforeseen consequences.

The overwhelming majority of *skin to skin* or *skin to fomites* contact *does not* transmit dangerous pathogens. Harmless microbial transmission and exchange virtually occur with every skin contact. This is the normal state of things. Handwashing decreases microbial counts as well as alters microbial population makeup and diversity. Handwashing therefore disrupts the status quo. The long-standing assumption that the benefits of handwashing always outweigh its downsides is only recently beginning to crack. Remember my "foam before you roam" adventure into ichthyosis? The question of how handwashing affects the hand, much more so than anything downstream from a mere change to the microbiome is likely too complex to fully analyze and comprehend. Each case is a unique example, and no statistical analysis can make a difference here as no individual is a statistic. Therefore, I suggest caution and discretion when practicing handwashing.

Discrimination and intention are key when using soap or any other cleaning practice on your skin. Handwashing is known to decrease (not completely prevent) the spread of infection in many settings. However, dangerous infectious pathogens are not the norm, especially in most Western households, specifically healthy households, which are the majority. Industrialized societies have eliminated or significantly decreased many sources of waterborne, airborne, and surface-related infection by extensive hygiene and decontamination practices such air filtration, water treatment, mechanized and detergent-mediated laundry, mechanized and detergent-mediated dishwashing, disinfection of fomites, as well as robust use of antibacterial and antimicrobial compounds in many applications.

Exposure to life-threatening pathogens has decreased accordingly, but with a price. Most microbes in the human environment are commensal or mutualistic. The definition of commensal according to the American Heritage Dictionary is "of, relating to, or characterized by a symbiotic relationship in which one species is benefited while the other is unaffected." The definition of mutualistic is "an association between two organisms of different species in which each member benefits." Traditionally, microbes on the skin have the arbitrary designation as either commensal per the above definition or pathogenic. This means people deemed them as either harmless, worthless sheep, or disease-causing wolves.

I suspect there are no truly commensal microbes, and every microbial element serves a unique purpose as part of the human ecological system, with the overwhelming majority being mutualistic. Starting in the early 2000s, the language around human-associated microbes started to shift becoming more nuanced, with the recognition the roles of microbes are virtually unknown and the beginning of discoveries of clear benefit for previously so-called "commensals."

Another caveat to understanding microbe-human relations was the traditional categorization of microbes by their physical appearance and biochemical properties determined by a limited set of tests. For example, a bacterium could be categorized as a gram-negative rod with resistance and sensitivities to a number of antibiotics, as well as other enzymatic properties. Those criteria helped in approaching microbes when relating to them as infectious agents, as well as for antibiotic treatment, offering little in understanding how microbes routinely interacted with the human ecosystem. Also, bacteria that could serve as commensal or mutualistic in one scenario, could turn pathogenic in another, depending on the host, sometimes without a clear explanation.

With more understanding of the importance of microbes, as well as improvement and refinement in analysis methods, the categorization is slowly shifting, becoming more nuanced, in stark contrast to medical establishment orthodoxy, and the public, still mostly classifying bacteria as either commensal or pathogenic, often using commensalism and mutualism interchangeably. I regard the definition of commensalism as a passive adjacent to parasitism, which, according to Merriam-Webster Dictionary, is "an intimate association between organisms of two or more kinds especially one in which a parasite obtains benefits from a host which it usually injures." Biology is transactional. No free lunches.

When examining the concept of hygiene, Roo Vandegrift and his colleagues proposed a clear and practical definition "those actions and practices that reduce the spread or transmission of pathogenic microorganisms, and thus reduce the incidence of disease."[59] The statement demonstrates an increasing specificity in dealing with the microbiome, microbes, clearly distinguishing and assigning value to different actions or practices in different contexts, reflecting not all microbes are the same, not all handwashing is of identical value, and certainly not all people and their life circumstances would benefit equally from handwashing. This highlights the need for establishing a personalized, nuanced, and intentional approach rather than a generic one.

Handwashing does not work perfectly for several reasons. First, handwashing does not generally eliminate microbes completely but temporarily decreases their numbers. This means there are remaining microbes quickly repopulating the skin. Second, while handwashing temporarily decreases microbial numbers on the hands, other surfaces such as a person's clothes, other parts of the skin, as well as fomites form a source to recolonize the hands by direct contact. Third, antibacterial soaps have no significant advantage over regular soap in preventing infection or reducing bacterial levels on the hands.[60] Fourth, over the past decade the concept of the "microbial cloud" was discovered, referring to a collection of airborne microscopic particles, including microbes surrounding the human body, which emit from the body orifices, as well as skin, hair, and clothes. So, no matter how effective handwashing is, there is always the microbial cloud to serve as a mode of transmission.[61]

Now, let's look again at handwashing. Hand hygiene practices are mostly non-specific, meaning they target commensals, mutualistic, and pathogenic microbes, which means handwashing can have significant unintended and presently largely unknown consequences. With the microbiome reportedly affecting domains such as cardiovascular and neurological health, we should be cautious in our advocating for handwashing and much more, so tread lightly with broader cleansing practices. So, where do we go from here?

One should determine the need for handwashing on a case-by-case basis, depending on the circumstances, type of product used for washing and the methodology. Having interviewed and examined many thousands of patients, I've met countless habitually washing their hands every time they pass by a sink or disinfecting their hands whenever they pass a dispenser. The era of COVID-19 made things much worse for countless people. This is clearly an indiscriminate practice of questionable value and can certainly cause significant skin damage in the form of dryness, irritation, damage to the microbiome, and beyond.

Handwashing has a proven benefit in decreasing the spread of infection, but we must consider whether this is applicable to our circumstances. First, handwashing in the healthcare setting, both outpatient and inpatient, has been of benefit, though not without adverse consequences. Healthcare settings are a special case where there is close and frequent human contact between microbiological strangers (not regularly sharing the same household or common spaces for extended periods of time) coming from different environments, with many of the participants afflicted with serious illness, infectious and non-infectious. In addition, the healthcare setting is a professional environment with special expectations and fiduciary responsibilities. Those implicit and explicit expectations compel healthcare professionals to wash their hands often to prevent spreading infectious microbes from one patient to the next and to their own colleagues. But what is the tradeoff or the negative consequences of handwashing?

Handwashing can cause skin damage and long-lasting modification of the microbiome, which could lead to an increase in potentially harmful microbes[62;63,64]. Carrie Zapka and her colleagues noted differences in hand microbiome with hygiene practices with swab samples but not with glove samples, demonstrating the limitations of the scientific method and the importance of choosing the appropriate, as well as diversified research tools.[65]

The food industry, the organized mass production of food for public consumption, is another category of settings requiring special care with regard to handwashing, with handling food sold to countless consumers. This translates to a possible infectious ripple effect where one contact handling food at its point of origin for distribution or sale could infect numerous people and cause widespread serious illness. Additionally, in the food industry there is frequent handling of naturally contaminated foods such as meat, eggs, dairy, and so on. So, handwashing after bathroom breaks, as well as after handling food is crucial, to prevent cross contamination, as well as promote personal health in the food industry.

On the home front, handwashing should be much more limited. Consider handwashing, especially in cases where household members are experiencing respiratory and gastrointestinal infection. Also, before preparing food and after handling food, in particular meat, eggs, dairy, and likely vegetables and fruit as well. Also, consider handwashing if you are a parent who changes diapers or cares for a sick child. However, limit same-household handwashing because household members come in close contact with each other, fomites, and animals around the home, as well as microbial clouds, meaning household members literally bathe in each other's microbes.

Breaking transmission completely is almost impossible. Life-threatening infections are relatively rare in the West. Bacterial overgrowth and mild infections, which make up most cases, are usually easy to manage, and recovery rates are high. And then there is the question of what handwashing does to commensal and mutualistic microbes? The answer is we don't know, not really. And more provocatively, what if we need exposure to so-called pathogens, to prime our immune systems or other benefits beyond our grasp? We don't know. The benefit to an individual by exposure to a subspecies of bacteria is impossibly complex to calculate. There are clues to the importance of pathogen exposure, for example David Strachan's report, which tied household size to increased rates of atopy.[66] The chronic and worsening atopic pandemic throughout the Western world closely ties to a variety of lifestyle changes, which decrease diverse microbial exposure.

Settings requiring frequent handwashing are the exception. While most people have no need to wash their hands indiscriminately and automatically, many do so anyway. It is redundant and likely harmful for a kid playing with his toys to then wash his hands because his helicopter parents want him to clean up. In fact, I strongly suspect the use of soap, synthetic detergents, and other products for the skincare of babies and children is harmful. Parents are under increasing pressure to raise their kids according to cookie cutter standards. This is an all-pervasive movement, driven by big government, big corporate, aided by activists[67] affecting child rearing, education, nutrition, general health, skincare, and beyond.

What was previously an already pervasive neurotic culture of handwashing, has exploded further with the COVID-19 scare with multiple hand washings with hot water (scalding the skin), mindless use of hand sanitizers further fueling an epidemic of skin disruption. The bottom line: use discretion when washing your hands.

The Wonderful World of Cleansing — Doubling Down by Innovation and Word Games

In the "Gentle Cleansing Fallacy" we discussed how the SIC creates new "gentler" products that are meant to address public concerns about their abrasive nature.

Other practices, which are harmful to skin integrity with no benefit are the use of mesh sponges, woven face cloths, scrubs, skin brushing, and hot water. Any product designed to abrade the skin, whether it's chemically, physically, or both, will damage skin architecture, integrity, and increase the need for externally provided skin protection, promoting the use of moisturizers.

Shampoos and conditioners share a similar relationship to abrasives and moisturizers. Shampoos generally are detergent-based products designed to cleanse or strip the hair and scalp of oils, as well as microbes. Conditioners are a category of products designed to control hair texture, specifically improve dryness and breakage. Shampooing the scalp has dubious health benefits, with exceptions when treating scalp conditions, e.g., dandruff, seborrheic dermatitis, psoriasis, and certain types of folliculitis. When in doubt, review the proper use of shampoo and the expectations with a dermatologist so you can agree on the right type of medicated shampoo, understand the improvement period, when to stop treatment, and how to determine whether the treatment is working for you. Even medicated shampoos create damage in their wake, frequently requiring compensatory conditioning.

Don't fall for the language games. No matter how many words you add to it, a detergent is still a detergent, an abrasive is still an abrasive, and use either with limits or not at all. If you *must* use an abrasive, use it as infrequently as you can, avoiding other elements that enhance the irritating effect such as hot water or washcloth. Less is more. Let's examine a few "unicorns" the SIC developed, look at the benefit they provide, and what purpose they serve.

Micellar water (MW) is a great example of SIC persuasion ingenuity, baked into product design. The term itself sounds sophisticated, scientific, credible, providing cover for essentially overpriced abrasive concoctions designed for makeup and oil removal, capturing them into tiny bubbles floating in water, which are micelles, acting as easily removable collectors of oils. The gentle promise of MW translates into their relative inefficacy, leading to their common leave-on use. Leaving MW on the skin forms a residue of weak detergents, as well as fragrance and other unnecessary ingredients, compromising tissue integrity and normal function.

Microbeads are tiny spherical objects, 5mm or less in size, many types of which are made of petrochemicals. The SIC has incorporated these elements into countless skincare products, including cleansers, scrubs, and even toothpaste[68] for many decades. They are a significant burden on the environment, entering the digestive tract of many animals, poisoning and suffocating them, as well as contaminating them as a food source throughout the entire ecosystem.

Legislation in the United States generously gave corporations years to eliminate microbeads from their products.[69] Data regarding SIC compliance with microbead legislation is unreliable, enforcement is sparse, and there is clear indication their use is still widespread[70], with little attention. Due to a combination of big money influence, politics, presumption of fiduciary responsibility, as well as ignorance, the deleterious effects of the SIC on the environment receive little coverage. So, the SIC gets to virtue signal and preach about environmentalism as well as other social justice concerns, and at the same time, it gets away with dumping pollutants into the environment with little accountability or transparency.

Snake Oil, Inc. — The Rise of Essential Oils, Vitamins, and Other "Natural" Ingredients

A category of so-called inactive ingredients, which I call the snake oil category has risen to prominence in the past few decades. The SIC and other industries add those ingredients, appealing by name, reputation, or branding, with a heavy hand and with an implied, yet seldom proven, benefit to the consumer. This is going to sound very blunt, but when you buy snake oil-infused products you're paying a premium on a deadweight buzzword at best or an actively harmful ingredient at worst.

Examples of snake oil are most essential oils, vitamins, ceramides, and peptides. These all have a great appeal, in part due to the perception anything natural or a vitamin being essentially beneficial and harmless, which is nonsensical. Nothing is categorically beneficial and harmless.

About Those Natural Ingredients...

First, most ingredients categorized as natural or healthy, such as vitamins, peptides, and ceramides, among others, require extensive processing, including chemical extraction, distillation, purification, modification, even synthesis. They are a hodgepodge of compounds and mixtures lumped together under an unspoken assumption of somehow being above other ingredients.

There's no serious evidence of the benefit of using most natural snake oils. Surely, some people reading this are asking, well what's the harm in using any of those chemicals and the short answer is: We don't know. There simply isn't enough information on the biological function, benefits, and adverse effects of topical application of essential oils, vitamins, peptides, ceramides, etc. Most of the reports are anecdotal and reliable research is hard to come by.

Chapter 5:
The Skincare Guide:
Buy Yourself Something Nice

After examining the formidable actors currently controlling the skincare narrative, let's put the power back into your hands — the individual. In the following chapters, we'll discuss how to truly care for your skin by forming a standard method to understand its basic needs and address them in the most cost-effective way, speaking basic *Skinese*. Work only as needed, spending fewer resources, exposing yourself to fewer potential side effects, while achieving the same or better results. Shed any unnecessary practices, while retaining the essentials. As we saw earlier, the time and money spent on skincare can compound to frightening amounts. It is my intention that you save as much of it as possible and spend it as you wish. Relax, buy yourself something nice, like a house, or whatever floats your boat.

A Word of Caution

"A man's got to know his limitations"
-Harry Callahan, Magnum Force, (1973)

As I've repeated ad nauseum, your skin is a highly complex organ. Managing persistent skin ailments is something best done under the nuanced and expert care of a board-certified dermatologist. This is not promotional advice. Most dermatologists will never have a shortage of patients. This is about knowing the limitations of your own knowledge and skill. Avoid digging yourself into a hole of unknown complications. If your skin condition persists with or without self-prescribed treatment, consult a board-certified dermatologist.

Shed Your Toxic Skincare Brands; Support Brands Working for You

In 2019, Gillette, a P&G subsidy, launched an ad campaign encouraging men to shave their toxic masculinity. In March 2022, P&G launched another ad campaign informing Chinese women their feet are five times more stinky than men's feet.[71] Both campaigns met with significant backlash. What do those campaigns mean regarding P&G's focus? Is it skincare products or social commentary?

One thing I've learned over the past few years: It's crucial to use skincare products manufactured by good faith actors. While it's impossible to know anyone's true intentions, we can judge them by their actions.

Considering social media, and other internet resources it's never been easier to determine your skincare manufacturer's focus. Before buying a skincare product, go to the manufacturer's website and social media. Check them out and see what they're about. Personally, I try to avoid companies engaged in virtue signaling and political statements as part of their brand, which invariably come at the customer's expense.

Moreover, with corporate mergers, acquisitions, and other misdirection, ownership of your favored brand may change or even not exist as advertised to begin with. There are reports many businesses claiming to be woman-owned fail the litmus test when further scrutinized[72] suggesting misrepresentation of the identity of business owners is common, sometimes amounting to fraud, betraying consumer trust.[73]

While personally I do not care about a business owner's identity, I understand how someone would. It simply is not a primary concern. What is of paramount importance to you is your own well-being and benefit from the products you purchase and use. If the identity of the owner is important to you, make it a secondary consideration to the value you derive. When I choose brands to use or recommend, I look at the product's quality and cost-effectiveness. My secondary concern is the brand's focus. If a company appears distracted by anything not directly related to their products, I know they are not investing their resources to fully serve their customers. It is a matter of physics. They have finite resources, generated through sales, meaning your money. They are a skincare company. If they are active in any other areas, they cease to be purely about skincare.

Skincare Brand Red Flags

Generally, corporate red flags are not irrefutable proof of wrongdoing but could indicate the company in question may become distracted from making the best products, helping guide you to look further. Those include but are not limited to the following:

Political or social commentary in advertising — My rule is if they're not advertising how their product directly benefits their customers, they're out. No preaching, no lecturing, no shaming, no fawning. Just tell your customers how your product works for them.

Political advocacy, virtue signaling on websites and other media releases — Much like advertising, I expect all company bandwidth to devote itself to their customers. If they have the resources to spend on political or social virtue signaling on their website, ads, pamphlets, and other media releases, they are shortchanging you from getting the best product for your money. Whatever they don't spend on your well-being, they spend on something *other* than your well-being. Here's a suggestion: If the executives using corporate funds for their favorite causes care so much, let them use their own resources rather than other people's money, namely yours.

Manufacturing their products abroad/foreign owned — There is nothing categorically wrong with imported products. However, besides buying a product that works *for* you, a locally crafted product means lowering energy expenditure, lowering premiums, creating jobs in your locality, state, or country, and greater accountability.

While becoming increasingly rare, there are still skincare brands putting their customers first. I lean not to recommend skincare brands, but rather a method of finding brand names working for you, literally. Vanicream is an example of a skincare brand whose politics I don't know from their website. I've had experience with Vanicream products for years used by numerous patients, and they manufacture first-rate products — effective, with few ingredients, and mostly affordable. Individuals or a small group own the company privately and are fairly small compared with the giants. Those are all great attributes for a manufacturer.

Cultivate Great Respect for Your Skin

Whether you believe God created us in his image or simply appreciate the infinite complexity of biology, know your skin is a miracle, a highly sophisticated orchestra even when unwell temporarily or chronically. However, with the right approach, there are basic concepts empowering you to understand your skin, its language, and provide answers as needed.

Understand Your Skin. Learn *Skinese*, Listen to It, Respond as Needed Only

How do you care for something as remarkable as the skin? Understand the basics, let it do its job, correct course when things go awry. Less is more.

How to Care for Your Skin: Principles Outlined

Caring for your own skin takes a principled and nuanced approach. There is virtually no room for categorical assumptions, or automatic behavior. Here are the hallmarks of best practice skincare.

Dump The Medicine Cabinet; Cultivate a Consolidated and Focused Approach

Ideal skincare is a transactional relationship: on point, intentional, and economical. Consolidate your actions and products you use. Keep it simple: one action and one product for each purpose. If you must cleanse, meaning use a detergent on your skin, choose one product.

If your skin requires moisturization, find the single best moisturizer and use it exclusively. Avoid using body area-specific products such as eye creams, face creams, hand creams, and so on. Those are redundancies, robbing you of money, time, and more.

Mind Your Own Skin

The most important traits to track are skin integrity and basic function. Well-functioning skin has a subtle shine to it, so subtle it may only appear as "not ashy," rather than gleamy. When the skin looks like this, the message in *Skinese* is "I've got this. Put your attention elsewhere." Healthy skin stands in contrast with ashy, or frankly dry skin, persistent redness, sores, as well as pimples.

From a sensory standpoint, healthy skin feels like nothing. One does not normally sense one's own skin unless the skin touches another surface, or when attention focuses on a specific body part. Ailing skin, such as dry, irritated, or broken skin persistently transmits sensations such as tightness, itch, burning, pain, "crawling ants," numbness, etc. These are signs of irritation or other issues requiring intervention.

There are cases where skin appearing intact (not dry or ashy) transmits abnormal sensations such as itch, burning, or numbness. This could be a sign of neuropathy or a systemic matter. Dealing with such issues can get very complicated, requiring a highly nuanced and personal approach.

Have Realistic Expectations

A common pitfall for skincare is unrealistic expectations about the degree of improvement, quality of change, or timeframe, often leading to disappointment and more mistakes.

Timeframes are one of the trickiest traps. Obviously, most people want quick and sustainable improvement of their skin issues. SIC propaganda creates an implicit expectation. For example, before and after photos of acne products create the impression of an overnight success.

So, what is the proper time period to expect improvement or resolution of a skin condition? It depends. Different areas of the skin, as well as different conditions respond within their own unique time periods. For example, the blushing episodes associated with rosacea may resolve within minutes with the right treatment or even spontaneously. Bacterial infections like cellulitis usually respond within hours or days with proper antibiotic treatment. Eczema usually starts responding within a few days to the correct treatment.

On the other hand, most cases of acne usually take six to eight weeks to improve convincingly and sustainably with appropriate treatment. Hair loss (alopecia) presents a wide range of timeframes, depending on the type of condition, with the fastest time for alopecia improvement being at least a few months. Nail disease is another category of conditions that improve slowly with the correct treatment. Then, there are individual tendencies of improvement, as well as personal circumstances such as aggravating factors, namely bad skincare habits irritating the skin, compromising its integrity and undermining the results of proper therapy. Therefore, it's crucial to have well-adjusted expectations and avoid adding unnecessary steps, wasting time, money, making matters worse.

Proper Retinoid Application

- When it comes to retinoids, their proper application and mitigation of potential side effects is crucial to a successful treatment.

- Because of their high efficacy, requirement of long-term use, as well as irritating nature, patients must uniformly apply retinoids as a tiny amount over a wide area. Unless explicitly advised by a dermatologist, patients must use topical retinoids only once daily at bedtime.

- For the face, apply a pea-sized amount. Dab the single pea-sized amount over the mid forehead, on the middle of each cheek, and the middle chin, then spread the product to cover the entire forehead, right cheek to right side of the nose, left cheek to the left side of the nose, the chin, and then spread this out even more overlapping areas of application.

- With dry, sensitive skin, moisturize your face before applying the medicine.

- Moisturize as often as needed.

- Avoid complicating your regimen with cleansing or other abrasive practices, unless your dermatologist specifically instructs you to.

Normal Skin Does NOT Need Moisturization

Most people do not need to moisturize their skin. The hallmark of normal skin is appearing intact without redness, pimples, sores, or flakiness and generating no persistent untriggered sensation. This is *not* numbness, but rather not sensing anything unless the skin feels appropriately stimulated by normal triggers like touch or temperature changes. Also, normal skin does not transmit any exceptional and stubborn sensations like tightness, burning, itching, or pain. If the skin feels like nothing, appears intact, free of redness, and dryness, it does not need moisturizing.

Letting go and leaving things alone is a challenge for many, especially with years or decades of indoctrination that you must do something. However, healthy skin already has enough moisturizing with the best fitting product possible, its own secret formula, a unique concoction the skin makes with such nuance and complexity no man-made product could ever match. I consider moisturizers a crutch or a prosthesis. People may use them temporarily or permanently, depending on the type of injury, but it never comes close to the real thing.

Oily or Mixed Skin is Usually a Self-Inflicted Problem

With a few exceptions, especially in healthy people, oily skin, and so-called "mixed" skin forms as a reaction to use of chemical or physical abrasion. This is a common concern on the face, with global excessive oil production or a mix of an oily T-zone (forehead/nose) and dry cheeks and chin. The best solution to oily skin is stopping abrasive skincare practices altogether. Use lukewarm water to wash your face and your oily or mixed facial skin will reset itself.

Discontinuing abrasive practices to an oily or mixed-skin face can be a leap of faith. For many this is a chicken and egg conundrum. In my experience, with a few exceptions, the chicken is the abrasive practice, oiliness is the egg. It takes about two to three weeks for oil production to reset and resume normalcy once the person discontinues the abrasion. This is the same for shampooing and oily scalp/hair.

Hot vs. Lukewarm Water

In my many years as a dermatologist, I have met countless people who use hot water, as in hotter than 105 degrees Fahrenheit or 40 degrees Celsius. That's hot as in fever hot. Fever causes many drastic biological changes to basic cellular function, protein structure, and activity for both human cells and microbial cells. In fact, fever helps killing various species of infectious pathogens. Hot showers or baths are harmful to the skin, scalding and irritating it to varying degrees, depending on the individual and other practices incorporated, e.g., soaping, scrubbing, brushing.

If your skin is already highly irritable, with conditions like hives or eczema, hot water will make your condition worse, sometimes immediately after exposure. Use lukewarm water for your showers or baths. Hot water may feel good immediately, but it compounds skin damage cleansing and scrubbing cause.

Cleansing

When it comes to cleansing, less is more. Use soap where it's needed for an explicit reason, and nowhere else. Why create changes and possibly cause damage where none is necessary? Use soap under the armpits, groin, and gluteal cleft, to address body odor and irritating residue. This approach has worked well for countless patients who have turned their dry, sensitive skin around by avoiding the very practice making them worse.

When it comes to babies and children, the less soap you use, the better off they'll be. Launch them off to a good start. Kids benefit from wide exposure to all kinds of microbes, as their immune system develops. They need "messy" play to become resilient to infection, as well as develop overall sturdy skin. My recommendation to the parents coming to my clinic is to use soap only as needed to clean off actual dirt and mud, as well as on the gluteal cleft to get rid of residual bowel movement.

When children reach puberty, they eventually start producing body odor. If their body odor bothers a child or teenager, they can soap the armpits, groin (not actual genitals) and gluteal cleft areas.

Disrupt the Antiseptic and Antimicrobial Craze

Unless serving a clear purpose, stop using any over-the-counter antibacterial and antimicrobial products. Eliminate disinfectant wipes, hand sanitizers, antibacterial soaps, antibacterial cleansers, antibiotic ointments, antifungal creams, antiviral topicals, or anything else meant to prevent infection or kill microbes. Your ability to prevent infection by using these products has limits, but the damage incurred by their indiscriminate use is incalculable.

Shampooing

Shampooing has little health value except for conditions such as dandruff or seborrheic dermatitis. Though those are not health benefits, some shampoos help condition hair by changing its texture, as well as scenting hair. I recommend you consider stopping shampooing altogether for three to four weeks, unless you're using it for any clear purpose other than cleaning. The scalp and hair will reset themselves, resulting in normalization of oil production. Now, some of you may be thinking: "This guy is crazy. I need my shampoo to achieve the right texture, so I can style my hair and give it the sheen that I like." Well, crazy aside, you're not wrong that some products can actually help achieve a certain desired look immediately. That being said, you may be able to have the look you like without shampooing. Healthy hair has a natural sheen. You may be pleasantly surprised by what your body produces for no extra charge. Regarding oiliness, remember the working paradigm: Shampooing is the chicken, and oiliness is the egg. So, give your hair and scalp a chance to reset. What have you got to lose?

For kids, there is no need to shampoo. Only kids with specific scalp conditions, such as dandruff, seborrheic dermatitis, or cradle cap may benefit from shampooing. Even then, I would focus on whether this condition bothers or affects the child negatively in any way.

If you must shampoo, by either force of habit or a feel-good benefit, consider lowering the frequency of shampooing from every day, to once every few days. Find your sweet spot for when you must shampoo to retain the desired effect, yet not overdo it.

Conditioning

Conditioners are a diverse group of products designed to make hair look and feel better, mostly making it softer or less likely to clump and easier to manage, i.e., style or shape. In cases where hair is exceptionally dry, tends to clump, or otherwise is challenging to style, conditioning may be of value.

If your hair is dry, damaged, or otherwise is challenging to style, investigate habits possibly damaging your hair. Specifically, if you shampoo frequently, use relaxers, or use any method applying dry and/or hot air you may be inducing your issues or worsening them. If you are using any hair damaging techniques and cannot help stopping them, consider using a conditioner to offset the damage.

If your hair is exceptionally dry and fragile, you can extend the time of application of rinse-conditioner to the scalp, enhancing its effect. Massage the conditioner into your hair and scalp, then cover your hair with a shower cap. Let the conditioner set for thirty minutes, then rinse. You're free to do whatever you like out of the shower while waiting for the product to further condition the hair.

Another option is leave-in conditioners. Using edible oils, such as argan oil, sunflower oil, coconut oil, or shea butter, is a great way of conditioning, especially in very dry frizzy hair, through adding emollience and occlusion.

Exfoliation

Exfoliation is a widespread collection of practices designed to strip the upper layers of the skin, having been around for at least thousands of years worldwide, dating back to ancient Egypt and traditional native American cultures, for example. There are over-the-counter, readily available forms of exfoliation and clinically administered forms, e.g., peels.

Some peels have benefits for addressing skin pigmentation and texture on a limited basis. Sometimes, exfoliation can help address skin spots or scars. However, users must evaluate the benefit of exfoliation for any skin issue on a case-by-case basis. The value of the procedure depends on the treated condition, the person's skin type, the technique used, and the method of use.

There's literally no evidence to support the benefit of exfoliation, "removing dead skin cells" as a regular practice. Exfoliation results in immediate injury to the skin and may lead to altering the properties of the skin. Exfoliation may have harmful effects on personal health and well-being, which are currently beyond our understanding. Avoid exfoliation as much as possible.

Scrubbing

Scrubbing is an enigma. Looking closely at any claim advocating scrubbing—the use of an abrasive element to physically buff the skin—you won't find anything remotely concrete to support its benefit. Scrubbing irritates and damages the skin. While there are some techniques using various types of injury to induce skin renewal, they have a wide spectrum of efficacy and users must tailor them to individual needs.

As with the gentle cleanser ploy, the SIC plays word games around scrubs, categorizing them as gentle, extra gentle, etc. Don't fall for this trick. Scrubs are abrasive by definition. Even if there are levels of abrasiveness, the practice has no proven benefit to begin with. Less useless is still useless. Therefore, I strongly recommend you do not use scrubs.

Toners

Another unnecessary and usually misunderstood group of products is toner. Toners are a redundant and likely harmful category of drying and irritating compounds, specifically various alcohols. A few toners contain alpha hydroxy acids (AHA), which can help in some cases of acne and photoaging. No one size fits all and AHAs do have side effects, namely irritation. Much like scrubbing and exfoliation, toners fall into the SIC Pepsodent Effect category. Unless you have a very clear reason for using a specific toner ingredient, don't use them.

Makeup Removal

There are endless choices for makeup removers. These products effectively emulsify and disassociate makeup along with attached skin elements. Like most other skincare products, manufacturers can attest they do not cause any clear and immediate harm. Again, this information is deeply troubling by what the definition of harm includes, or rather by what it *does not* include. We do not fully understand the damaging effects of products like makeup removers. Even so-called gentle makeup removers still disrupt the skin barrier. Don't fall for the word game.

So, what can you do? Some makeup products can be easily and safely removed with water. If that's the case, use water. If the makeup is heavier or designated as water-resistant, my recommendation for makeup removal is to use edible plant-derived oils such as sunflower oil, argan oil, or coconut oil. Massage the oil into your hands, apply to the face, and wipe the makeup away with a cotton ball, or a dry makeup removing pad. Then rinse the residue with water, with whatever remaining oil on the face acting as a natural emollient/occlusive. While most people tolerate all three oils well, a few patients reported irritation with coconut oil.

Makeup Removal Done Right

Whether it's my preferred powder makeup, paste, or liquid, all products are nearly completely removed using this simple, cheap, and moisturizing method.

Load about half a teaspoon sunflower seed oil, argan oil, or coconut oil onto your hand, then massage the oil onto the entire face.

Wipe the oil/makeup mixture away using a cotton ball, or a dry disposable makeup remover pad.

Rinse your face with lukewarm water.

Pat (not rub) residual water with a towel.

Your face will remain covered with a thin residue of oil, which acts as a moisturizer. While I've never encountered sunflower seed oil, or argan oil irritating anyone's skin, I know sometimes, although rarely, coconut oil can irritate the skin.

Peels

Peels are a mixed bag. Like toners, there are some conditions possibly helped by certain types of peels. Peels also come with possible side effects such as irritation, blistering, and discoloration. Severe and long-lasting side effects are not common and usually associate with inadequate patient screening, poor technique regarding timing of application or product deactivation. Peel expertise requires extensive training and the consequences of using peels without expertise can be disastrous.

Some peels can help specific cases of melasma and other forms of skin darkening. Some peels can improve severe and widespread sun damage. An expert with clearly demonstrated efficacy must match to and apply a specific peel for the condition. Avoid using peels as a self-help tool or a generic "good for you" and "what's the harm" approach.

Cosmetic Masks

There are several categories of masks: (a) sheet masks; (b) peel-off masks; (c) rinse-off masks; and (d) hydrogels. Their supposed purpose is a mishmash of fiction and fact. As a generality, there is little evidence to support any use for masks. Detoxifying or nourishing are not actual functions of any skincare product, let alone masks, but SIC-speak for a nonspecific "good for you." My advice: Avoid using masks. If there is some medical necessity for using a mask and there is clear evidence to support its use, then go ahead and use it as directed.

Serums

Serums are expensive, very popular snake oil. Traditionally, the word serum is a term referring to a category of biologically formed fluid complexes. It does not refer to anything concocted in a lab or a factory. So, frankly, I see it as a term deliberately hijacked and exploited to give a false aura of scientific credence to a dubious synthetic product. Consumers and less discerning skincare professionals abuse the term unwittingly or the SIC use it intentionally to launder and greenlight the use of worthless yet pricey products.

Cosmetic serums are emulsions which are runny in consistency, mostly comprised of water, alcohols, preservatives, emulsifiers (including those alcohols), and artificial coloring. There are various mentions of pseudoscientific terms around them. Categorically, treat any claims made about cosmetic serums with the utmost suspicion. Don't believe the hype and save your money for something nice.

Vitamins

Unlike serums, masks, or toners, which have limited value, possibly harmful, vitamins — small molecules vital to various biochemical processes — are of great value with several caveats. First, vitamins are a heterogeneous category arbitrarily lumped together by scientists, physicians, and others for various reasons. With such diversity in this category, lumping vitamins together can lead to confusion about their benefit.

Science and its capabilities to clarify biology have been and continue to be grossly overestimated. For example, vitamin E, sometimes referred to generically as tocopherol, classically viewed as an antioxidant participating in cellular reduction-oxidation (redox) homeostasis, is not simply a single molecule. It's a complex of molecules and metabolites with roles extending well beyond balancing reduction and oxidation. This is highly misleading, and we do not fully understand the role of the tocopherol complex in redox homeostasis or in any buzzword process. Beyond our limited understating of biochemistry, our understanding of human biology is ever changing, growing, and evolving. Therefore, addition and promotion of so-called vitamins in skincare products are troubling.

Vitamins aren't simply good for you. It's a matter of the form of the vitamin, the circumstances, the quantities and how you take the vitamin. There is a time and place for everything, a context in which one thing is necessary and another is redundant or even harmful. With our limited understanding of topical vitamin application, I classify vitamin additives to skincare as either one of four categories:

1. Snake oil/promotional mention with unknown quantities of the ingredient sprinkled into the mix to create a buzz and FOMO, promoting sales and use of the product, likely being the main impetus behind all vitamin additions/mentions, even if there is an additional secondary benefit.

2. Adding preservatives — tocopherols, tocopheryls, or ascorbic acid (vitamin C) — to skincare products as antioxidants/preservatives.

3. Skin conditioning — tocopherols can function as emollients, and possibly occlusives, though I doubt they're better than a superb emollient/occlusive such as petroleum jelly or sunflower oil, which incidentally contains small amounts tocopherol.

4. Long-term use benefits, likely through induction of gene expression, this type of benefit is observable and quantifiable and requires weeks or months of consistent use. Vitamin A-related molecules are the most used category to induce sustainable changes such as increased collagen production, resulting in plumper and smoother skin. With over-the-counter retinols or retinoids, most of which are prescription grade in the U.S. (except adapalene), the effects are more noticeable, yet still fairly subtle, requiring several months of consistent application.

The most encountered side effect with topical vitamin application is skin irritation, and in some cases allergic reactions. This is particularly common with retinols, retinoids, and can also occur with tocopherols.

With a few exceptions the benefit of topical vitamin application in skincare is mostly nebulous and may result in skin irritation. I recommend consulting a board-certified dermatologist before purchasing expensive products under false claims. Also, do your own research. Go beyond the blogs and testimonials. Look for contrarian views. If so inclined, examine the scientific literature. While retinoids, even adapalene, which is sold over the counter in the U.S., can be very helpful to skin texture, complexion, and other features, make sure this is the right approach for you. There are variations in retinoid strength, utility and side effect profiles, and they simply don't universally fit any skin type. I advise against using retinoids while pregnant or trying to conceive.

Chapter 6:
The Moisturization Guide:
Work with Your Skin

Working with your skin, rather than SIC slavery, is the key to good skincare. Your approach must be straightforward, attentive, and consolidated.

- Aim for simplicity with products and practices. The product or practice you're using must meet the declared goal in the most cost-effective way, meaning, the safest or least harmful, most effective, and cheapest product wins.

- Pay attention to your skin and learn to evaluate its needs on an ongoing basis, from one area to the next with the full understanding these needs keep changing as they should.

- Consolidate your approach, meaning strive to complete any skincare goal with as few steps and products as possible. This means getting rid of many redundant products and stopping the dreaded capricious "product rotation." The key word is consolidation. Consolidate, consolidate, consolidate.

Whatever you pick, keep it simple. Choose a single product and learn to apply it from head to toe on an as-needed basis. The scalp can be an exception. There is no such thing as an area-specific moisturizer, only arbitrary labels designed to maximize profit, so don't fall for this ploy. In my practice, I recommend several categories of moisturizers from which you can choose. The common denominator for most products I endorse is they are safe[74] to use anywhere on the body, as well as occlusive, meaning oils. Those are the most effective, least irritating, and in many cases most affordable products. Creams and lotions are generally inferior to a great ointment or balm.

Oiliness requires a nuanced approach to application. Oily products go a long way with tiny amounts. A drop-sized amount can be enough for each body area, e.g., the arm, the shin, the face, and so on. Proper application while avoiding smearing and staining requires attention, artfulness, and practice. However, this is immensely beneficial and saves you time and money.

Dry and Sensitive Skin

Dry and sensitive skin is *Skinese* for "Pay attention. Stop what's not working. Help out conservatively. Carefully observe."

Persistently dry skin from head to toe must first be an abrasion free zone. Do not make things worse by adding insult to injury and discontinue any chemical or physical abrasion including hot water. If the issue persists, moisturize the affected area appropriately, with a few exceptions, which I'll address separately.

Top Moisturizers

When considering what makes a great moisturizer, I look at several factors, including the level of protection it affords, durability, safety, and lastly texture. Occlusion affords protection. While the hygroscopic properties of a moisturizer, or its ability to draw water to itself, can be of value, ultimately an oily layer needs to protect water content, so it does not evaporate.

Durability, how long a product stays on the skin, matters since it determines the frequency of application. The longer a product lasts, the less work for you. Safety is complex, as I previously discussed. Some factors helping in determining safety are low likelihood of irritation, or allergenicity, as well as limited effects on the microbiome. So, it was important to consider product purity as far as content of occlusive elements to other ingredients. Texture is important to the application experience, determining the pleasure in applying, as well as what happens after you apply: excess residue, runniness, etc. We end up with a short list of oils with a limited number of ingredients.

Petroleum jelly is an occlusive, which is highly effective, safe, and affordable. You can apply it from head to toe. Contrary to urban legends, petroleum jelly does not clog pores, meaning it is not comedogenic, and you can safely use it on the face. Just take it easy with the amounts. Why take it easy with the amounts? First, it doesn't look good. Too much petroleum jelly and your skin can look too shiny with chunks of the compound. Second, too much petroleum jelly will stain clothes, sheets, furniture, and more. Those two issues alone lead to much of the aversion to using petroleum jelly or other greasy moisturizers. One must know how to artfully and effectively apply a moisturizer.

Plant oils such as coconut, sunflower, and argan oil can work as moisturizers. One recurring issue with them is their low viscosity, meaning they are runny. Use them if you like, just watch the amounts. *Do not use* olive oil; it can be comedogenic and promote yeast overgrowth on the skin.

Shea butter can work well as a moisturizer. Most shea butters are highly viscous at room temperature and can be grainy. So, if you choose to use shea butter, use small amounts and if the product is grainy, warm it up between your fingers for a few seconds before applying it to the skin to avoid abrasion.

Compounded vegan balms combine a few oils for optimal viscosity and smoothness. My recommendation for products in this category emphasizes a minimal number of ingredients, safety, and U.S.-made. Whenever evaluating a product, go beyond the front label claims and closely examine the ingredient list. You'll be surprised by how many products claiming to be vegan or giving the impression they contain nothing but natural ingredients incorporate less than desirable and often redundant ingredients.

I personally created my vegan balms to minimize the number of ingredients, making sure they all work for you with three edible ingredients or less. Find the latest at drbibiorganics.com/skincare.

Remember, for some of the simpler single oil products – the edible grocery store version is a terrific option. Coconut oil and sunflower oil are widely available in most food markets.

Proper Moisturization

Unlike the automatic, tedious, and redundant "everybody needs to moisturize" approach, which is literally universal at present, properly moisturize exclusively, as needed. A common complaint regarding moisturizers, especially occlusives, is staining clothes, sheets, and furniture. Here's what to do.

- Oily or consistently normal skin does not need moisturizing; simply leave it alone.
- Dry, sensitive skin requires moisturization anytime it gets dry or, even better, just before.
- Proper application of a moisturizer is meant to put a "subtle shine" on the skin, nothing more.
- Apply *only* as much as needed for restoring the skin's subtle shine. With greasy moisturizers or occlusives, apply a drop-size amount to a body area such as the forearms, shins, hands, or a similar sized area. Spread this amount evenly over the skin, until there is nothing but shine without a hint of a residue.
- Nighttime is the most important time for moisturization since one cannot moisturize while sleeping.
- Especially with dry room air in closed, air conditioned, or heated areas, consider adding a humidifier to your bedroom, adding moisture to the room air and slowing down TEWL.
- Be sure to clean your humidifier regularly to prevent mold.

How Often Should You Moisturize? Be Your Own Skin Whisperer. Anticipate, Evaluate, and Calibrate Your Skincare

Inadequate moisturization, not knowing when and how often to moisturize, is common. How often do you need to moisturize? The answer: The skin will tell you, in *Skinese*. With dry skin, you must moisturize no matter how many times a day. Some people's skins feel satisfied with once or twice a day, while others require more. If the number of times you need to moisturize seems excessive to you, consult a board-certified dermatologist to address possible skin irritation, infection, or other causes of flaky skin.

Bedtime Moisturization

Bedtime is the most common pitfall, especially for people with dry skin. Consider this. When you go to sleep, you'll spend many hours with your skin losing moisture to the room air while you can't compensate. This gets worse in air-conditioned or heated rooms combined with low humidity.

Therefore, moisturizing before bedtime for someone with dry, sensitive skin is crucial. Apply the product over problem areas as you would any other time. For people with very dry hands or other limb parts like the shins, an occlusive wrap such as gloves or plastic wrap can be helpful during exceptionally dry episodes.

Control Room Air Humidity

Air humidity is a key factor in determining how much moisture you lose to the room environment. Therefore, if your bedroom is dry, add a humidifier. This will decrease the strain on the skin and make your moisturizing efforts more effective.

Scalp and Hair Moisturization

Persistently dry scalp, as well as frizzy, fragile hair needs moisturizing. If you can use a conditioner, whether it's a rinse conditioner or a leave-in conditioner, be sure to apply the product to your scalp and hair. With exceptionally dry hair, try applying a rinse conditioner for extended periods of time – about thirty minutes under a shower cap, then rinse for an augmented effect.

People with exceptionally dry, frizzy, and fragile hair may benefit from applying oils to the scalp. In my experience, the best three oils are coconut oil, sunflower oil, and argan oil. Applying any type of oil requires a nuanced approach, using only as little as needed or risking drippy excess, staining of clothes and sheets. So, when applying any scalp oil start small and build up gradually to get the right amount needed.

Face Moisturization

The face is an amazingly sturdy area of the skin, naturally rich in oil glands, meaning usually well moisturized. The T-zone, the forehead and nose, is usually oilier than the cheeks, chin, and perioral (around the mouth) areas. This difference can become starker with frequent abrasive treatment of the face. If you experience persistent dryness or sensitive skin on the face, moisturization goes a long way.

Load a tiny drop-sized amount of moisturizer on your index finger, dab tiny amounts on the forehead, right cheek, left cheek, and the chin. Then using your three middle fingers, massage the moisturizer onto the skin covering the entire area of application. The entire forehead is one area. Spread the product from the right cheek to the right nose, left cheek to the left nose, then around the mouth and chin. You must spread the product out as far as it goes until you can no longer spread it, as thin as possible, forming an effectively micro-occlusive layer on the surface of the skin. Get the benefit of the product while not wasting it or ending up with excess product on your skin, which can look unnaturally shiny and can stain fabric.

Lip Moisturization

Lips are also particularly sturdy but can get drier than the rest of the face. Saliva residue, as well as lip balms, and other products can irritate the lips. With dry lips, remember, the skin will tell you how often it needs moisturizing. Many don't realize most lip products are practically petroleum jelly diluted with redundant and possibly harmful ingredients, including dyes, fragrance, essential oils, plant extracts, vitamin E, and more. Save time and money and stop using overpriced, compromised products. Either petroleum jelly, shea butter, or shea butter-based moisturizers I mentioned would work well as lip balms, applied as a drop-sized amount as often as needed.

Arms and Legs Moisturization

Arms and legs can be exceptionally and persistently dry, especially the shins. Because they are large sized areas, many feel tempted to use large amounts of moisturizer, leading to dissatisfaction with any residual product and oiliness. The best way to moisturize a large area like a limb is to take a drop-sized amount of product (any of one of the products above) and spread it as far as possible. In most cases, a tiny amount is enough. Remember, your goal is putting a "subtle shine" on the skin, with anything more making no positive impact and possibly staining your clothes, sheets, or furniture.

Hand Moisturization

Hands can be exceptionally challenging to moisturize; they can become persistently dry and irritated. Often, we must wash our hands or treat them in other ways, making matters worse. In addition, fingertips, or web spaces (the skin folds between fingers) can become fissured, forming painful cracks. Fissures are a problem besides simply being painful, posing a persistent disruption of skin integrity, allowing elements to seep in, forming a vicious cycle of irritation.

Whenever possible, protect your hands preemptively when doing potentially irritating work. Wear gloves when working with solvents, petrochemicals, washing dishes, or any other activity irritating the hands. No matter how sturdy your skin is, don't take it for granted or willingly abuse it. Even the most resilient skin has a breaking point, challenging to reverse. Don't get there in the first place.

Dry hands need moisturizing consistently and repeatedly, especially after handwashing, or other wet work followed by drying. With hands encountering many surfaces, conscious moisturizing of problem areas and avoiding intact areas can mitigate staining workspace surfaces and other fomites. So, moisturize dry and cracked areas, avoiding healthy areas. Pay attention and always act out of meeting need, clearly stated in *Skinese*, rather than autopiloting.

As I mentioned before, nighttime is a window to significantly compromised moisturizing. For dry irritated hands, gloves can help seal the moisture and possibly a topical medication onto the skin, allowing better occlusion.

Painful fissures can benefit from sealing with either liquid bandage or acrylic glue. Make sure you're not allergic to acrylates, avoiding compounding your skin irritation. The solution can't be worse than the problem. Sealing hand fissures can help break the vicious cycle of compromised skin integrity and allow the skin to heal with proper care. A word of caution: Most cases of chronically cracked skin need active treatment with powerful prescription medications, so consult a board-certified dermatologist.

Foot Moisturization

Feet are challenging to moisturize, requiring a wholly unique approach. They are a relatively dry area on top, but the bottom of the foot is a completely different breed of skin, often sweaty and moist. Dryness treatment on the top of the foot is usually easy as I described above. However, dryness on the bottom of the foot may not be dryness at all, but flaky skin related to athlete's foot, which moisturizing can worsen. I'll address athlete's foot shortly. When in doubt, consult a board-certified dermatologist to clarify the cause of your "foot dryness."

Flaky Skin That Is Not Necessarily Dry Skin — Special Cases

While dryness causes most cases of flaky skin, there are other causes of flakiness. This is important because those conditions do not respond to moisturization as expected, with some even worsened by it.

Dandruff

Dandruff and its more inflamed relative seborrheic dermatitis are conditions thought to occur when the skin becomes sensitized to a common yeast naturally found on most human skin. Dandruff presents as non-adherent white flakes on the scalp, sometimes associated with itch or more rarely burning. Seborrheic dermatitis can be more widespread, affecting the eyebrows, the ears, the sides of the nose, the chest, the armpits, the groin folds, and genitals.

Because of the connection to yeast, many cases of dandruff and seborrheic dermatitis respond to antifungal compounds, usually in shampoo form. Over the counter options include shampoos containing zinc pyrithione, selenium sulfide, and ketoconazole. There are prescription shampoos as well, including ketoconazole (in a higher concentration than the over-the-counter option) and ciclopirox. Treating dandruff requires persistence, using the shampoo once daily or once every other day for a few weeks until the condition is under control, then backing away, using the shampoo once a week or about to maintain the results. I recommend adding a conditioner to shampooing to offset dryness. An antidandruff conditioner, available commercially, may eliminate the need to moisturize.

Very dry hair makes frequent shampooing impractical. If your hair is frizzy and fragile or you simply don't want to shampoo, consider an antifungal cream application twice daily directly to the scalp. The advantage of using a leave-in antifungal is focusing treatment on problem areas, controlling the amount used, and possibly adding moisturization.

If your scalp condition does not improve within a few weeks, or you're experiencing redness, flakiness, or pimples with hair loss, seek dermatology evaluation immediately. This could be one of several very serious conditions, including psoriasis, lichen planopilaris, skin lupus erythematosus, etc.

Tinea Versicolor

This condition manifests as oval or round flaky spots, usually appearing on the chest and back, which is the result of overgrowth of a yeast naturally found on the skin. The spots don't tan as well as the rest of the skin, leading to unsightly hypopigmented or lighter-color blotches. Certain people are more prone than others, likely due to genetics. The treatment is either by topical antifungals, used much like the antidandruff products discussed previously, or in more severe cases prescription antifungal pills.

Athlete's Foot

Athlete's foot is a fungal infection of the bottom of the foot, and between the toes. The most common form is flaky skin on the bottom of the foot, mistakenly leading people to moisturize the affected area. The problem: Fungus thrives on moisture, making athlete's foot worse, so it's crucial to keep the feet dry, including after showering, adding cornstarch powder into socks before you wear them. Also, changing socks daily is a good idea to prevent reinfection.

Athlete's foot requires active treatment twice daily with antifungal creams, either over the counter clotrimazole, or prescription grade ciclopirox and econazole. There are other antifungal products available over the counter as well.

The trouble with athlete's foot goes beyond distinction from dry skin. There are other conditions possibly mistaken for athlete's foot requiring additional evaluation. Those conditions include but are not limited to erythrasma (a bacterial infection), psoriasis, dermatitis, and, rarely, skin cancer.

Normally, athlete's foot significantly responds or resolves within two to three weeks of treatment in most cases. So, if you decide to treat your athlete's foot on your own, have a clear endpoint where you decide whether this treatment is working. If your treatment is not effective, consult a dermatologist.

Tinea Corporis

Tinea corporis (TC) is fungal infection or ringworm of any part of the arms (not hands or fingernails), legs (not groin, feet, or toenails), as well as trunk. TC usually presents as circular flaky red areas whose center is often less prominent giving the impression of a ring. Unfortunately for the inexperienced diagnostician, there are several other conditions appearing similar whose management is remarkably different, sometimes even diametrically opposed to the treatment of TC. This means treating suspected TC without a clear and certain diagnosis can make your condition worse. Moreover, curing TC frequently requires a combination of topical and prescription oral antifungals. If you're certain you have TC (an expert made the diagnosis), treat with a topical antifungal twice daily. Response time to correct treatment is usually a few weeks. If the condition does not improve or becomes worse — redder, flakier, more painful, burning, or spreads — this is a red flag that should prompt you to consult a dermatologist.

Chapter 7: The Nail Guide

Nails are a highly complex organ, often traumatized by day-to-day life, as well as a variety of grooming practices. You can't avoid life, but you can tone down grooming, which damages the nails. Excessive buffing, trimming of the cuticles, applying nail polish, as well as removing nail polish, are a few traumatizing practices. Nail grooming practices have their place. However, simplifying them is worth considering. Nails and cuticles benefit from moisturization, using the same products previously mentioned.

"Not All Nail Fungus": Dystrophic Nails — A Special Note

Dystrophic nails or abnormal nails are very common. Also, realize there are many reasons for which nails can be abnormal, with different changes often meaning different nail disease. This is a wide and complex range of changes, which in most cases require a highly specialized professional to make the distinction. Most people, including many physicians dismiss any abnormal nail as "nail fungus." However, this is frequently a misdiagnosis, leading to wrong lengthy treatments, ranging anywhere from a few months to many years.

Consider the following, with the correct diagnosis and optimal treatment, fingernails normally take anywhere from three to six months to respond noticeably. Toenails can take anywhere from six to nine months. That may not look like complete resolution of the problem but can look improved. This is a long period of time to invest, so we must diagnose correctly. We can pivot to a different treatment in case the first one fails, knowing what condition we're treating.

Treating many patients suffering from a variety of nail issues has taught me humility. I've stopped counting the number of patients who came to see me confident they have "nail fungus" only to realize they're suffering from a completely different condition after a proper workup. Many patients I evaluated went through years of treating their nail conditions until disillusionment set in and brought them in for a second opinion. Generally, there are no great over-the-counter remedies for any common conditions causing nail dystrophy, including nail fungus, warts, psoriasis, lichen planus, alopecia areata (yes, a condition leading to hair loss as well nail dystrophy in some cases), and growths, benign and cancerous.

Here is a non-exhaustive table of a few nail conditions illustrating the complexity of nail dermatology. The list is meant to empower you. Some of you may be asking how does almost always sending me to a dermatologist empower me? With wisdom and knowing one's own limitations comes great power. We cannot always do it on our own. Nail dermatology is one of those areas where great expertise and nuance is necessary, at least to get you started with meaningful care.

The Wonderful World of Nail Lesions – Don't Try to Diagnose This at Home			
Condition	**Appearance**	**Clues**	**Diagnosis, Treatment & Bonus Points**
Nail fungus or onychomycosis	Thickened nails; grey, yellowish, or light brown discoloration; subungual debris	Usually, several nails involved Athlete's foot often present	Diagnosis with bedside KOH. Fungal culture or pathology take longer and are more expensive. Treatment with oral antifungals; less common is laser ablation. Resolution takes long months with correct treatment.
Nail warts or onychopapilloma	Thickened nails; grey discoloration; subungual debris.	May involve several nails	Diagnosis may require a nail biopsy. Liquid nitrogen or topical agents such as imiquimod or 5-

The Wonderful World of Nail Lesions – Don't Try to Diagnose This at Home			
Condition	**Appearance**	**Clues**	**Diagnosis, Treatment & Bonus Points**
			fluorouracil. Treatment is challenging and can take many months.
Nail psoriasis	Thickened nails; grey, yellowish, or light brown discoloration; subungual debris. "Oil spots." Nails may shed in severe cases.	Plaque psoriasis	The doctor can make a clinical diagnosis of psoriasis, although it may require a nail biopsy when in doubt. Treatment ranges from topical steroids/vitamin D analogs, intralesional injections, systemic medications. Long months to clear with appropriate treatment.
Nail lichen planus (LP)	Roughening of the nails, splitting	LP of the skin, oral cavity, genitals	Diagnosis is possible if LP is present elsewhere. May require a biopsy when in doubt. Treatment with topical, intralesional, or systemic steroids. Other systemic medications may also work. Scarring and permanent deformity of the nail matrix are possible.
Onychomatricoma	Thickening, discoloration and raising of a nail.	Usually involves a single nail.	Diagnosis is possible with a nail biopsy. Treatment is surgical removal. This is a

The Wonderful World of Nail Lesions – Don't Try to Diagnose This at Home			
Condition	**Appearance**	**Clues**	**Diagnosis, Treatment & Bonus Points**
			benign growth of the nail matrix.
Squamous cell carcinoma	An often-painful nodule with or without ulceration of the nail/digit; can lead to thickening of the nail, discoloration, and subungual debris.	Involves a single nail/digit	Diagnosis is possible with a nail biopsy. Treatment can consist of local surgery, or in cases of lymph node spread and metastasis may require chemotherapy, biologic therapy, and radiation therapy.
Malignant melanoma	Brown, black, red, or pink discoloration under the nail bed with or without a nodule, possibly leading to thickening of the nail plate; may lead to ulceration; Often, lesion, including discoloration may spread to surrounding skin on the digit.	Involves a single nail/digit	Diagnosis is possible with a nail biopsy. Treatment can consist of local surgery, or in cases of lymph node spread and metastasis may require chemotherapy, biologic therapy, and radiation therapy. Hutchinson's sign refers to discoloration spreading to the digit, often over the cuticle. In early stages, can be confused with subungual hemorrhage or bruising under the nail bed.

Workup is straightforward, starting with an interview, examination, and appropriate confirmatory tests. Nail fungus diagnosis can sometimes be made with a quick test called potassium hydroxide (KOH) prep. It involves scraping debris (or "gunk") from underneath the nail plate if there is anything to scrape, laying it on a glass slide, adding KOH solution and examining the preparation under microscope, which is possible in minutes in a clinic. If the KOH prep is negative and there is still a strong suspicion of nail fungus, a culture is a good idea.

If the KOH prep (and/or fungal cultures are negative) and a visual diagnosis is not reliable, a nail biopsy is the best diagnostic approach. This requires skill, a willing dermatologist, and motivation on your part to go through the procedure. This will provide a bottom line, specific treatment options, and help set realistic expectations for the results. It is not magic but is the most reliable way of figuring out the best approach for your condition. If you or a loved one are suffering from dystrophic nails, do yourself a favor and see a board-certified dermatologist to properly manage your condition.

Not nail fungus

Patients consistently show up with "nail fungus," that is a nail or nails that stand out for whatever reason, ready to treat it as such. They're often surprised that this may not be nail fungus at all and sometimes something quite unexpected.

When Monica (real name withheld), a 35-year-old actress came to see me, she was certain she had nail fungus on her right index fingernail. "I'm ready to treat it and get rid of it." she said, pointing to a pink bump the size of a carraway seed under the fingernail. When we discussed her issue further, Monica mentioned she's had this for about two years. She's tried to treat it with some antifungal creams and even tried a few months of prescription topical nail fungus medication. My thoughts as I was examining Monica's spot is that this did not look like nail fungus at all but was certainly worth investigating. I advised Monica that we would have to get to the bottom of what's causing her nail problem and perform a nail biopsy, not quite what she expected. After discussing the procedure with her, Monica agreed to go through with the biopsy and we were both glad she did. Her so-called nail fungus turned out to be a malignant melanoma in-situ, a superficial type of skin cancer.

Monica needed surgery, not antifungal treatment. She was lucky she made a point of getting a skin exam, despite having no previous history of skin cancer and pointing out something that was barely noticeable and required treatment, just not what she expected. This is an extremely rare example of "nail fungus" turning out to be something that's potentially life threatening.

Legendary musician Bob Marley, died of metastatic malignant melanoma which started under his big toenail. Marley initially thought this was a soccer injury. However, when the lesion persisted, a doctor biopsied it and diagnosed malignant melanoma. It is reported that Marley opted for a more conservative treatment approach and declined to treat aggressively by amputating the toe. He eventually died of metastatic melanoma in Miami, Florida on May 11, 1981.

Now, obviously most nail dystrophy is not skin cancer. However, it is helpful to get clarity before making assumptions about nail changes. Clarity can make the difference between cure or persistence of the problem, and in the rare event between life and death.

Chapter 8: Genital Skincare Guide

Skincare of genitals is a charged issue considering the significance and controversy of sex, as well as the wide range of emotions brought on by it, including shame, guilt, and fear. If most people consider skin dirty almost as an oversight, genitals are commonly consciously associated with undesired "dirt," "filth," "disease" and other buzzwords prompting "special care," such as abrasion, scenting, and other grooming practices, like hair removal. Focused attention coupled with shame, guilt, and fear create a barrier to seeking medical attention when things go wrong.

Genital grooming for both women and men has exploded over the past few decades. The most common forms of grooming are hair trimming and hair removal by waxing, laser, electrolysis, etc. Less common practices include hair dying or bleaching, piercing, injectable enhancements, laser surgery, other device interventions, and plastic surgery, e.g., labiaplasty in women and circumcision or to the contrary foreskin restoration in men.

Skincare routines for genitals range from washing with a detergent and hot water, through use of additional abrasives, as well as application of scenting, and moisturizing elements. Due to shame, guilt, and fear, many take treating issues arising over their privates into their own hands (no pun intended.) The availability of a wide range of over-the-counter products purporting to treat anything from yeast/fungal infections (e.g., miconazole) to symptoms such as itch or pain (e.g., benzocaine) fuel this behavior. Much like other skincare issues, online access to numerous resources created the illusion of a wealth of knowledge and agency leading to an exaggerated faith in the ability to precisely diagnose and treat without training or fundamental understanding.

In my many years of treating patients suffering from genital disease, one of the most common issues I've encountered is excessive grooming and care leading to irritation or worsening of an ongoing problem: an infection, an irritation, or even cancer. In many cases, those very practices are at the root of the problem or making it worse. Most problems arising over the genitals relate to irritation of the skin. In some cases, the irritation is idiopathic[75] and in some it relates to a chemical irritant, a physical abrasive, or an allergen applied to the skin.

Much like the face, the genitals are generally very sturdy relative to other areas, with inherent robust glandular function, moisturizing, and repair capabilities. As such, genital skin, as well as the adjacent vulvar mucosal surface in women and foreskin in men, can put up with a lot of abuse. But every person has a breaking point.

My advice: Tread lightly. Avoid use of detergents directly on the genitals, meaning penis and scrotum in men and labia, vaginal opening, and vagina in women. Avoid hot water, high pressure streams, abrasives such as washcloths, sponges, scrubs, brushes, or loofah, and unnecessary moisturization.

While I understand the urge many feel to trim, shave, or otherwise remove pubic hair, I advise against it. Pubic hair has a protective function and removing it can unnecessarily irritate the skin, make you more vulnerable to infection, and be associated with painful intercourse in women. If you insist on shaving, trimming, waxing, or any other hair removal technique, keep in mind this is an irritating, abrasive practice. As such, I recommend choosing the gentlest hair removal method, as well as compensatory moisturization.

For wiping purposes, avoid using baby wipes or other wet wipes because they are very likely infused with preservatives and even fragrance. Use soft three-ply toilet paper or a wet paper towel lightly soaked in tap water.

If you experience any rash, pimples, bumps, or any other new development over the privates, my advice is to see a board-certified dermatologist for an initial evaluation before treating. You'd be amazed at the complexity and variety of conditions arising over the area. It is certainly not a one size fits all.

So, if you are not sure, do not treat with whatever is available. Conditions affecting the genitals have a special stigma associated with them, with many sufferers assuming they have a sexually transmitted infection. The benefit of distinguishing genital conditions from sexually transmitted conditions is immense from both a perspective of morale and peace of mind, as well as health and proper care. Seek professional evaluation and management to clarify your genital condition.

Regarding strong odors emanating from the vulva or the groin; they are *usually* a sign of microbial overgrowth, inflammation (such as psoriasis) or both. There are other less common causes of bad odors. Do not try and treat this on your own.

Treatment timeframes for genitals vary between a few short days for certain cases of inflammation and infection but can stretch out to weeks or months, depending on the condition. Be sure to set your expectations with your physician.

When you find yourself in a hole...

When I first met Jane (real name withheld), a 28-year-old woman, she thought her life was over. Jane was traveling from her home country in the Middle East to the United States when she started experiencing a mild itch over her private parts. On her first layover as her symptoms were persisting, she decided to do something about them. She used an over-the-counter cream called Vagisil, which she has used before for the occasional itch. Vagisil, commonly used for vaginal itch, contains two potential allergens, benzocaine and resorcinol. She also added hot water soaks and resorted to scrubbing the area to "clean" the skin further.

After a few days of using Vagisil and "cleaning," by the time she got stateside, Jane's symptoms intensified, and she began noticing foul odor and redness over the area. Thinking this was a yeast infection, she bought a second medication, Monistat, containing miconazole, an antifungal compound, which is also a potential allergen. After a few days of combination treatment with the two creams, the situation became noticeably worse.

At that point, Jane's vulva was red, swollen, itchy and painful. She also noticed a clear smelly discharge. She saw her primary care doctor. After examining her, Jane's doctor was deeply concerned about a compound infection involving fungal, bacterial, and herpes simplex virus, obtaining cultures from the area and prescribing systemic antifungals, antibiotics, antivirals as well as recommending daily soaks with benzoyl peroxide, an antibacterial wash. The doctor suggested that Jane continue all her over-the-counter creams.

The following day, Jane's vulva "exploded" per her description. The area was beefy red, raw, extremely painful, and she could barely walk. She went to see her gynecologist who thought that this could be an irritation and recommended that Jane use over-the-counter hydrocortisone cream. The gynecologist concluded that between her and the primary care doctor everything there was to do was done and decided to consult me.

When she came to see me, Jane was obviously very upset and thought that she would never be able to have sex again. And by the way things were looking and the multiple failed attempts to treat her condition, I could see why she would think that. When I examined Jane, I diagnosed her with erosive vulvitis.

The name implies irritation that is so severe the skin breaks apart. My conclusion was that it was likely a combination of steps she and some of her providers took that resulted in an exacerbated situation. First, her description of her initial symptoms was consistent with irritation. Irritation of the skin is a complex condition to treat, but the principles are simple. Remove the offending agent, if possible, which in her case may have been related to prolonged travel, and if the symptoms persist, treat with an anti-inflammatory medication, usually a steroid.

Using a product like Vagisil did not address the underlying cause or the irritation and likely worsened her irritation. When things got worse, Jane thought she was dealing with a yeast infection and used miconazole, making her irritation more severe. To make matters worse, but consistent with "common sense" and "couldn't hurt" mindset, Jane began to "clean" the area. This consisted of elements adding more physical and chemical irritation by means of hot water, scrubbing, and making things worse with benzoyl peroxide washes.

As her irritation was getting worse, her gravely worried doctor used what's called "the shotgun approach." Fire in all directions hoping to hit something by adding treatments for a variety of suspected causes. Now, while her systemic medications likely did not make her condition worse, those are not without their own associated risks, including widespread allergic reactions and microbial changes leading to intestinal disease called pseudomembranous colitis, for example.

My approach was simple, and this simplicity took significant amounts of great mentorship, training, and experience geared to treat this problem precisely. Jane and I agreed to discontinue all of her previous practices: no cleaning, no scrubbing, no hot water, no creams, no pills. I recommended that she practice brief lukewarm soaks of the area, five to ten minutes without any soap or antibacterial compounds. I also recommended that she apply petroleum jelly to the area, a non-reactive and greasy protective element. As an aside, application of petroleum jelly soothes severe irritation almost immediately by occluding the skin from outside elements. It is not a complete solution, but it's a good start.

Next, we agreed that the irritation was so severe it was only going to respond to systemic steroids. Topical steroids were not going to cut it. The skin was too damaged. I treated Jane with an intramuscular injection of triamcinolone. Jane showed up for her follow-up appointment a week later with the irritation almost completely resolved. The area appeared mostly normal with no swelling, little redness and no discharge. Most importantly Jane was symptom-free. She experienced no itch or pain. Needless to say, she was a happy camper.

When I look back at this story, whose severity is unusual, I can see many points of failure in the management of Jane's case. I believe all failure points stem from a lack of education and experience, breeding reflexive no-questions asked approaches. This is at the heart of a much larger issue: the death of appreciation for true and earned expertise.

Not surprisingly, Jane's cultures were negative, meaning they detected no infection by a virus, bacteria, yeast, or fungus.

So, when you find yourself in the metaphorical hole, stop digging. Stop your abrasive practices to allow the skin to reset itself, catch up and resume its normal and desired function. Should things not improve, see a dermatologist.

About That Itch...

As a dermatologist who sees patients for issues affecting the genitals, I have the opportunity to hear many stories of patients who come to see me as a last resort after long weeks, months, years, and sometimes even decades of a persistent problem. In many cases, the women and men I counsel are embarrassed, ashamed, and often had no idea what medical professional, if any, could make sense of what they're experiencing.

While starting out as a specialty whose focus was on genital disease, dermatology has shifted its attention dramatically to other skin concerns, especially in the past fifty years. There are many considerations to this shift. Many are uneasy about the association with genital disease and the implication of sexually transmitted disease or infection (STI). As an aside, the majority of problems affecting the privates are not sexually transmitted or infectious. Some are uneasy about discussing those problems with patients and some are simply interested in other areas or subjects. There is only so much one can put on their plate. The bottom line is dermatology is no longer synonymous with venereology (STI), or with other issues affecting the privates, which are predominantly not infectious.

With the vast majority of issues arising on the genitals and the perianal area, there are simple steps people can take to improve their situation. Some of those steps are purely about a more focused approach and doing no harm as illustrated in the genital skincare guide.

However, in many cases a conservative approach will not be enough. Here are a few conditions affecting the genitals board-certified dermatologists should definitely evaluate and manage, and in some cases, with the help of our colleagues in OB/GYN, urology, pediatrics, internal medicine, and primary care.

Before we go into the list, keep this in mind. If you are experiencing a persistent problem over the genitals or perianal area, whether it's redness, flakiness, shiny whitish areas, sores, bumps of any kind, or symptoms such as tightness, burning, itch, pain, or any other persistent sensations, you need a doctor to evaluate you. If any changes or symptoms persist for more than a few days, let alone weeks, seek professional help.

Many a time, you'll be surprised things can improve easily. You'll get clarity and even if the news is not good, at least you'll know what you're dealing with and have a plan to address the issue. On many occasions I've had people come in expecting the worst and coming out with some great news. Don't live in doubt. Get the clarity you deserve.

Conditions affecting the genitals

Lichen sclerosus/balanitis xerotica obliterans — Lichen sclerosus (LS) is a chronic, inflammatory skin condition of unknown cause that can affect any body part of any person but often affects the genitals (penis, vulva) and is also known as balanitis xerotica obliterans (BXO) when it affects the penis. LS is not an infectious condition and can initially present as itchy red spots on the privates that persist over weeks or months, eventually turning into shiny ivory-white firm areas. In its most severe forms, LS can cause permanent scarring destruction of the areas it affects, specifically narrowing of the vaginal opening and/or the urethra, obliteration of the labia and clitoris, and in men scarring changes to the penis and urethra. Additionally, chronic LS associates with a higher risk for SCC developing over the affected areas. While most patients are adults, this condition can affect children, particularly girls, so awareness, early detection, and management with the help of a dermatologist is vital. This could literally save your life or the life of a loved one.

LS is sometimes mistaken for a yeast infection and erroneously treated with antifungals leading to delayed appropriate treatment.

Lichen planus — Lichen planus (LP) is a chronic inflammatory condition that affects the skin, nails, hair, and mucous membranes, including the mouth and the genitals. It has multiple forms of presentation and can cause itchy reddish-purplish, or lacy-white areas, as well as painful sores on the genitals. LP is not an infection. Much like LS, LP, especially the erosive variant can lead to scarring of the vulva, deformity, and development of SCC. Due to the severe and chronic nature of LP, early detection and management with a dermatologist is crucial.

Zoon's balanitis and vulvitis — ZB or ZV are a chronic inflammatory condition of the penis or the vulva, presenting as reddish areas, which can sometimes itch. It can be a source of great embarrassment. This is not an infection. With its chronic nature, ZB can wax and wane over time.

Psoriasis — a chronic inflammatory condition that can affect the skin from head to toe (including genitals), the nails, and in some cases the joints, known as psoriatic arthritis. Psoriasis is not an infection. On the privates, it often presents as reddish areas with or without silvery-white scale, which can sometimes itch or burn and sometimes is asymptomatic. Psoriasis can sometimes look like tinea cruris.

Seborrheic dermatitis (SD) — a chronic inflammatory condition affecting the skin, especially over the scalp and face, but can also affect the chest, armpits, groin, and genitals. SD is not an infection. On the privates, it can present as pinkish-reddish scaly areas, which can sometimes itch or burn and sometimes is asymptomatic. SD can sometimes look like tinea cruris.

Dermatitis — an irritation of the skin that can affect any area of the body, including the genitals, depending on circumstances. Either an irritant or an allergen coming in direct contact with the skin usually causes it. It is not an infection. Dermatitis can present as itchy reddish flaky areas, but in severe cases can cause severe swelling and even sores of the affected genitals. Dermatitis can sometimes look like tinea cruris.

Folliculitis — an inflammatory category of conditions, specifically involving hair follicles that can affect any area on the body, including the face, trunk, scalp, genitals, and buttocks. Folliculitis can be infectious or non-infectious and can sometimes be a challenge to diagnose and manage.

Hidradenitis suppurativa (HS) — a chronic inflammatory condition affecting hair follicles that can occur under the armpits, under the breasts, and on the groin/genitals causing painful pimples, lumps, boils, and in more severe cases, scarring of those areas. HS is not an infection, and a dermatologist must diagnose and manage it.

Syringoma — a type of a small benign skin-colored growth that can erupt, presenting as multiple bumps over the affected areas, mostly the eyelids, but can also affect the armpits, abdomen, chest, neck, scalp, or groin area, including genitals, in a symmetric pattern. Syringomas are not infectious but can sometimes be mistaken for warts by the untrained eye, especially when appearing on the genitals.

Sebaceous hyperplasia — bumps comprised of oil glands that can appear on many body parts. When they affect the genitals, they are Fordyce spots (FS). FS are not infectious and can sometimes look like warts or molluscum contagiosum.

Genital warts (GW) or condyloma acuminata — GWs are verrucous or flat growths affecting the genitals, and their color may vary, tan, brown, gray, white, pale yellow, or pinkish red. GWs are infectious and certain types of human papilloma virus (HPV) cause them.

Seborrheic keratosis (SK) — benign (non-cancerous) flat or raised light tan, brown, black, or pinkish skin lesions. SKs are not infectious. They are round or oval, and often feel like a barnacle or a scab from a healing wound, ranging in size from a few millimeters to several centimeters in size. SKs can sometimes look like GWs, so it's important to consult a dermatologist to make the distinction.

Angiokeratomas — tiny benign growths of blood vessels that can present as reddish to dark purplish bumps and can affect the genitals, usually the scrotum and labia majora in middle aged and older people. Angiokeratomas are not infectious.

Candidiasis — an infection caused by a type of yeast called candida (there are many different types) that can affect the mouth, different parts of the skin, the nails, and genitals. On the genitals candidiasis can present as reddish flaky or moist areas, and in more severe cases can cause sores. When affecting the vagina, candidiasis can cause a milky discharge. Candidiasis is very common, but doctors must distinguish it from other conditions affecting the area, especially if it hasn't responded to anti-yeast medication.

Cancer — several types of cancer can and do occur on the genitals, specifically SCC and MM, although other types, including BCC, can occur as well. Cancer can present as a painful sore, a persistent pimple, or a pigmented nodule or a blemish, which can sometimes grow, change in color, or shape, or form sores after first detection. Because the privates are a source of embarrassment for many, sometimes cancers of the genitals can go undetected for a long time. It's important to be aware of the possibility of developing cancer on the genitals and self-examine regularly, as well as get regular checkups and see a dermatologist if you suspect anything.

Intertrigo — a Special Category

The following section is a word of caution not to go at it alone. Treatment of intertrigo can get dicey very quickly. I encourage you to take what's written here so you can have an informed conversation with your dermatologist when evaluating your condition. Except for either stopping all product application to the area or switching your applied skincare products to fragrance-free and dye-free deodorant/antiperspirant and observing for improvement, I advise against attempting blind treatment on your own. Here's why.

Intertrigo is a highly complex group of conditions occurring in areas where the skin folds onto itself causing redness, flakiness, "cuts," and symptoms such as burning, itching, and pain, etc. Those include the armpits, groin, privates, under the breasts, and buttocks. In people who are overweight, intertrigo can involve abdominal folds. In many cases, intertrigo consists of several overlapping distinct conditions, making evaluation and subsequent management exceptionally challenging. The main issue with intertriginous areas is physical friction, as well as being very susceptible to chemical stagnation and abnormal microbial overgrowth.

Intertriginous areas are naturally moist, whether it's normal sweat production, excessive sweat, normal or abnormal secretions that occur when those areas become inflamed or infected. This forms a challenge in treating any problem arising over the area because it is rich in surface irritants. Naturally and normally produced sweat prompts use of antiperspirants, which can potentially irritate the skin and induce microbiome changes.

Intertriginous areas naturally produce body odor, especially in puberty. Most body odors are not very strong and are well tolerated. However, as a society we have gone way past the point of this consideration, resulting in a pervasive norm of automatic washing/cleansing of intertriginous areas, as well as widespread use of perfumes and deodorants, carrying a similar potential as antiperspirants, used to decrease sweat production.

People tend to thoroughly wash the area *before* coming in for an evaluation. Washing the area, even the night before your visit to the dermatologist, decreases surface elements that could be creating the problem in the first place. Whether it's fungus, bacteria, or other elements, the more of them are on the surface the easier it is to make the diagnosis in the clinic or. in some cases. by sending out tests. I strongly recommend not washing the night before or the morning of your dermatologist appointment. Remember: The reason for your visit is not to look good or spare the doctor's feelings but to find out what's going on and get better.

While intertriginous areas are chaotic, most people do very well and spend a lifetime with no issues whatsoever, serving as another testament to the miracle of the human body. As I mentioned earlier, those areas are so sensitive, when things go wrong, they can suffer from a single condition or from several overlapping conditions compounding each other. Let's review a few examples.

Tinea Cruris — "Jock Itch"

Tinea cruris (TCr) or jock itch (JI) is a fungal infection of the groin area, sometimes extending to the genitals and buttocks, appearing as red, flaky itchy areas with an undulating border, which can be asymptomatic, itchy, burning, or even painful. This can be very challenging to treat as fungus thrives on moisture, naturally occurring in the groin area. Another challenge of treating TCr is extension into hair follicles, often making topical treatment inadequate to fully eradicate the infection. TCr can overlap with other conditions, specifically bacterial overgrowth, as well as erythrasma, which is a form of superficial bacterial infection and confused with other conditions such as dermatitis or psoriasis.

Diagnosis is easy to do in a clinic within five to ten minutes using a KOH prep. If you're using antifungals, know that they significantly decrease the sensitivity to this test. My recommendation is to evaluate suspected JI with the help of a board-certified dermatologist to determine the right approach. If you decide to treat your JI on your own, be sure to limit the treatment to no more than two to three weeks, beyond which you must seek a dermatology consultation if your condition has not significantly improved.

If the groin area is exceptionally moist, thoroughly dry after showers, and use powder-grade cornstarch to soak up residual moisture. This is good practice regardless of infection status since it can help prevent infection and decrease irritation. Mild cases of TCr may respond to topical antifungal creams applied twice daily over the affected areas, such as clotrimazole, terbinafine, etc.

Erythrasma

Erythrasma is a common superficial bacterial infection occurring in armpits, groin, in-between toes, as well as other skin folds, often indistinguishable from TCr, as well as other intertriginous conditions. Erythrasma requires evaluation by a dermatologist, using a special type of light device called a Wood's lamp, inducing a special coral-red fluorescent glow. Remember not to wash the night before or the morning of your visit so you don't render the test worthless. Erythrasma is easy to treat with topical prescription antibiotics, which should show a response within weeks.

Bacterial Overgrowth

Bacterial overgrowth is a serious issue in susceptible individuals, creating a tendency for irritation over the affected area, as well as possibly serving as a reservoir for infection elsewhere, with Methicillin-resistant Staphylococcus aureus (MRSA). The suspicion for bacterial overgrowth can arise with overlapping issues as well as with irritation that appears to be resistant to conventional treatment. Diagnosis of bacterial overgrowth requires swab cultures, obtained in a clinic, usually taking a few days to brew, with results, including an antibiotic sensitivity report targeting treatment.

Seborrheic Dermatitis

Beyond the scalp and face, seborrheic dermatitis (SD) can affect intertriginous areas and can cause issues like any other form of intertrigo. The diagnosis is challenging, demanding a high level of expertise, possibly requiring a skin biopsy.

Treatment may comprise of topical antifungals, topical steroids, other topical anti-inflammatory medications, or a combination thereof. In very severe cases, treatment can include systemic medications.

Inverse Psoriasis

Psoriasis is a highly versatile condition that can affect any part of the skin and be associated with systemic issues such as psoriatic arthritis. Much like SD, this can present a diagnostic challenge, and ultimately may require a skin biopsy to determine.

Treatment may consist of topical steroids, topical vitamin D analogs, other topical anti-inflammatory medications, or a combination thereof. In very severe cases, treatment includes systemic medications.

The correct diagnosis of psoriasis is especially important because it can associate with serious systemic issues such as arthritis, a tendency for metabolic syndrome, and other conditions requiring scrutiny.

Dermatitis — Irritant or Allergic Contact Intertrigo

Intertrigo dermatitis or *irritation* is one of the most challenging conditions to treat in the skin folds, often with multiple active factors fueling the issue. Direct chemical irritation, allergic contact reaction, microbial overgrowth, and a combination thereof can cause dermatitis of the skinfolds.

Much like the previous conditions, this requires high level expertise to diagnose and manage. In many cases, the patient must withdraw an unrecognized offending agent whether it's a cleanser, a cosmeceutical, or a medicated topical. Active treatment may involve topical steroids, other anti-inflammatories, and in severe cases require systemic therapy.

Chapter 9:
The Hair Guide

The Importance of Hair Professionals

Hair professionals: barbers, hairstylists, hairdressers, and others are the frontline of early detection of hair loss or skin cancer of the scalp and adjacent areas. I consider their keen eyes, expertise, and involvement crucial to have your back, inform you of any abnormalities, and urge you to seek medical attention. A well-trained, responsible hair professional is worth his or her weight in gold. When your hair professional informs you of any unusual findings — pay attention.

Hair Thinning/Alopecia

Hair thinning or alopecia[76], the clinical term, is a common, serious problem. Another term used interchangeably with hair thinning is hair loss. Yes, alopecia *means* hair thinning, any hair thinning, specifically, unintentional hair thinning for any reason is alopecia. About half the population, both men and women, suffer from some form of alopecia. Much like nail dystrophy, alopecia is not a single disorder but a diverse category of many conditions. Much like disorders of the nail, the scalp responds slowly within many months under ideal conditions with correct treatment. Assumptions regarding the nature of the hair loss and attempts at generic treatments lead to wasted time, incur undesired side effects, and, most seriously, further hair loss, possibly irreversibly.

Nebulous generalizations regarding hair loss are a goldmine for the snake oil market. Unsuspecting consumers buy countless mostly bogus solutions. The answer: evaluation by a board-certified dermatologist, preferably someone devoted to management of scalp conditions.

To get an idea of how complicated hair loss can get, let's look at some facts. There are several categories of hair loss: scarring and non-scarring, inflammatory and non-inflammatory, acute (short term, which could still last months) and chronic (progressing over years). It gets even more complicated. Those categories include over ten different conditions. There could be an overlap of two or more types of hair loss. Also, non-scarring alopecia may or may not be reversible, depending on type, duration, and management.

Another element making hair loss challenging is when patients seek medical attention after months, years, or even decades, with often irreversible damage. I've heard many reasons for delaying care, including not having realized this is not "normal," thinking this is simply part of getting older, not knowing who to turn to for medical attention, or unsuccessfully attempting a variety of home remedies without a clear definition of effective treatment or a timeframe. Many types of hair loss do not readily and quickly respond to treatment. Management of hair loss requires experience, nuance, and patience. Even then, treatment may fail to achieve the desired outcome.

The good news: There are effective treatments for many types of alopecia. However, there is no one size fits all. So, do not let some layperson lead you astray by the hollow promises of the supplement industry, or the hair loss industry, starting any treatment without consulting with a board-certified dermatologist. In my experience, evaluation, establishing a clear diagnosis, and making an informed decision regarding care with the right expectations make all the difference. Do not take shots in the dark, denying yourself a chance at proper care.

Reversible Hair Loss

There are several types of reversible alopecia, some requiring active management, while others recover spontaneously.

Telogen Effluvium

Telogen effluvium (TE) is a condition leading to abrupt scalp-wide hair shedding and thinning, which can be very scary for anyone. Frequently, TE appears three months following a significant life event: death in the family, childbirth, major surgery, major illness, or starting a new medication to name a few. Many cases *cannot* trace back to any event. Most cases stop and reverse themselves within six to nine months with no treatment. Rarely, TE can become chronic, progressing for a year or more.

Alopecia Areata

Alopecia areata (AA) is an autoimmune condition targeting hair follicles, and sometimes nails. The most common form appears as circular bald spots on the scalp and the beard area with more *severe* and *rare* cases affecting eyelashes, eyebrows, and other body areas. The good news: Most cases are reversible with proper care, which usually consists of steroid injections into the affected areas. Most patients tolerate the treatment well and experience regrowth within a few months.

Severe and resistant cases are rare. However, many of those too are manageable, with varying degrees of success. Vitamin D deficiency can be associated with AA and contribute to disease severity and resistance to treatment.

My ponytail is thinner!

In many cases hair thinning starts small. In fact, the beginning of hair loss can be so subtle, it's tempting to think it's in your head. — no pun intended. A common line I hear in the clinic is "I know I have a lot of hair, but this isn't my baseline."

Kaylee (real name withheld), a 26-year-old bartender, is sitting on the exam table anxious to hear what is causing her hair to fall out. "It's like my ponytail has thinned by half. I used to have more hair than anyone I know," she tells me. After a brief discussion and examining her scalp, the diagnosis is clear. Three months before her big tsunami of hair thinning, Kaylee had major surgery, a bowel resection due to diverticulitis. She spent two weeks in the hospital and was slowly getting back to her old rhythm when clumps of hair coming out with combing, hair washing, on her pillow, as well as a frighteningly noticeable widening part width sidetracked her. Where her head was previously covered with lush thick hair, she could now see her scalp.

Desperate to do something, Kaylee started using a hair supplement from a reputable company, containing biotin among other vitamins. After a few weeks of patiently waiting for the shedding to stop and the hair to grow back, it was time to see the dermatologist. Fortunately for Kaylee, I'm the bearer of good news. Kaylee has TE. Her hair will stop this craziness all on its own and grow back to its old happy thick self, maybe not as fast as we'd like. But it will happen.

TE is the most common cause of "ponytail thinning." This type of hair is usually short term, whole scalp, and reversible, turning around in six to nine months. Some cases lack a clear trigger, some start about three months following a significant life-altering event, such as surgery, major illness, child delivery, starting or stopping a medication, etc.

Some cases of TE are chronic, lasting years, sometimes related to vitamin deficiencies or endocrinological disorders, with most cases lacking no clear cause. Most importantly, hair loss comes in many different forms. Therefore, especially with something as tricky as hair loss, I recommend seeing a board-certified dermatologist to manage your condition and address any questions.

In a few cases, TE can be related to systemic underlying issues such vitamin D deficiency and thyroid imbalance. Those cases can become chronic. Some cases of chronic TE are inexplicable. In those cases, treatment is challenging and regrowth fickle.

Progressive Alopecia

Unfortunately, many types of hair thinning are progressive, and many irreversible without and often despite proper treatment. Some may slow down or stop with appropriate management.

Androgenetic Alopecia (AGA) — Pattern Hair Loss

Whether it's male pattern or female pattern hair loss, AGA is the most common type, affecting an estimated 50 percent of men and women. While this is non-scarring, usually progressing slowly, do not let it fool you. It is extremely challenging to manage, requiring dedication, tenacity, and handling expectations as most cases *are not* fully reversible.

Lichen Planopilaris (LPP)

When it comes to scarring hair loss, permanently obliterating hair follicles, LPP and closely related *frontal fibrosing alopecia* (considered a subtype) are the most common. LPP can appear abruptly and cause immense permanent scalp damage, so a prompt diagnosis and management are imperative. Even with a quick response, LPP is notoriously difficult to control.

Central Centrifugal Cicatricial Alopecia (CCCA)

This condition is mostly exclusively diagnosed in women of African descent and less frequently in men of African descent, though men may be under diagnosed due to overlap or confusion with AGA.[77] CCCA causes scarring, i.e., permanent, hair loss over the central scalp or vertex, sometimes spreading outwards to involve a larger area. The cause for CCCA is unknown, but recent studies showed certain gene mutations can predispose to developing it. Once CCCA has progressed and "burnt out," it is *mostly irreversible*. In my experience, most people suffering from CCCA seek dermatology evaluation at very advanced stages, which is tragic, especially since many cases are potentially stoppable early on or even prevented.

Education, early detection, and action can make a world of difference. Because CCCA is associated with inflammation around the hair follicles, I recommend paying close attention to hair grooming practices irritating the scalp, decreasing, or stopping them altogether. Scalp irritation leads to sensation of tightness, itch, or burning, as well as skin changes such as redness, a purple hue, lighter discoloration, or flakiness.

Pay attention to those signs, acting fast to avoid *any* practice irritating your scalp to prevent CCCA from developing. If you suspect CCCA, seek medical care by a dermatologist *immediately*. Take proactive measures. Persistent irritation of the scalp, meaning symptoms lasting days, weeks, months, or years, is *not* a normal or desirable condition. If you are suffering from *persistent* symptoms of irritation over your scalp, despite stopping suspect practices or never having implemented them, seek medical attention as soon as possible. This will clarify the condition affecting your scalp and help treat it.

Other Forms of Progressive Hair Loss

Due to the incredible complexity of the nature and treatment of hair loss, I will mention several other types of progressive alopecia and end the discussion here. What we've covered so far is enough to realize this is no trivial matter and requires expert medical care as early as possible. Other types of progressive hair loss appear in cases of lupus, psoriasis, seborrheic dermatitis, traction, folliculitis decalvans, etc.

I hope this book spreads further awareness about the usefulness of dermatologists in managing hair loss. Not noticing one's thinning hair is very common. This is due to several possible factors, including continuous grooming with no breaks, masking early-stage thinning, as well as denial. The assumption of thinning as a given aging process is somewhat reasonable; hair can thin *slightly* with aging. However, significant hair loss is not normal, and therefore requires diagnosis and management.

Hair Vitamins, Formulas, and Complexes Are the Worst

People spend a lot of money, time, and other resources for a glimmer of hope. Dealing with hair loss, especially abruptly and rapidly, is a big deal. I've met countless patients suffering from hair loss, with many having already started some form of treatment, mostly on their own. Many of those self-treatments include hair supplements, commonly a mixture of vitamins, minerals, plant extracts, animal extracts (e.g., collagen, fish oils), amino acids, hormones and so on, claiming to benefit hair growth. Taking those products is plain wrong and can cost you dearly. Here is how. Hair loss is not a single entity or disease but rather a highly complex category of often overlapping conditions with a variety of causes. The dermatologist must evaluate each case of hair loss separately, and managed appropriately, address specific causes with a clear set of expectations and timeframe.

Treating any individual case of hair loss with an arbitrary shotgun approach of a formula or complex ignores the singularity of the case, often lacks clear definition of the type of hair loss treated and the issue addressed with the supplement, as well as missing clear expectations regarding aspects including but not limited to results of hair density, hair quality, and timeframe.

Most cases of hair loss are decidedly *not* related to a known or demonstrable vitamin deficiency and will not respond to supplements in a meaningful way. If there is a specific nutrient or vitamin deficiency, a dermatologist must evaluate and treat at the right dose, monitor to ensure you reach treatment goals.

Most of the ingredients in hair formulas do not directly promote hair growth. Treatment not fit for your type of hair loss and with unclear expectations can lead to disastrous consequences: wasting time, money, and losing hair, often irreversibly. I've seen countless patients who independently took hair supplements for alopecia. I have not met a single patient who took the appropriate vitamin type or dosage befitting their condition, or anyone who derived any clear benefit from those products. In many cases, self-treatment delayed proper evaluation and management.

Moreover, the vitamin and supplement industry is loosely regulated, with evidence-based and regulatory guidelines for putting products together almost nonexistent. This manifests as a wide variety of products capriciously designed with a mishmash of ingredients at arbitrary quantities and quality that is extremely difficult to verify,[78] raising serious safety concerns.

From the hundreds of people I've seen in the clinic, the majority who successfully treat hair loss with vitamin supplements are invariably cases of TE. This means reversal of hair loss in those cases would have happened with or without supplements. Correlation or coincidence are not causation. So, what were those patients doing presenting for evaluation if their hair loss responded to treatment? There are two main categories. One is a fortunate category of patients asking for a second opinion with an already improving condition.

The second category of less fortunate patients are those who have had a reversal of their telogen effluvium while taking supplements, subsequently developed a second type of hair loss that did not respond to supplements as expected. Counseling and managing hair loss in the second category can delay significantly due to the illusion of the utility of supplements. Patients in this category may come in after months or even years of faithfully taking supplements due to their past success, falsely associating spontaneous reversal of their previous hair-loss with self-treatment.

Otherwise, hair supplements are very helpful — for the good people who produce, promote, and sell them. As far as benefit for hair growth, I would categorize hair formulas as harmful products generically recommended without knowledge of your specific condition, with no clear benefit, often leading to delay in diagnosis and management by a professional.

Do not buy or use hair supplements either to preemptively prevent hair loss or to treat an ongoing problem.

Consult a dermatologist to diagnose your condition, determine the appropriate treatment, and set your expectations accordingly. This requires years of experience from your dermatologist. You may end up hearing some things you did not expect or want to hear, but at least you'll have clarity and understand what they can do. If your condition is related to a specific vitamin deficiency, your dermatologist may recommend and even prescribe vitamin supplements. Let's look at specific single vitamin supplements used to treat hair loss.

Biotin

Biotin is probably the most popular supplement associated with hair health and treating hair loss. Many patients come in using biotin, confident it's good for them. Obviously, their predicament has not improved in association with biotin, or else they wouldn't have come to see me. Despite a very long track record for recommendation and used for hair loss, there is no convincing body of evidence to support wholesale recommendation of biotin for hair health or hair loss, with studies being too small, lacking rigorous diagnostic criteria, or adulterated by conflict of interest to name a few issues. There may be some utility for biotin supplementation in cases of biotin deficiency and hair loss, but once again the evidence to support such intervention or provide any standardized guidelines is virtually nonexistent. Therefore, I am against any generic prescription of biotin as a remedy for hair loss or a promoter of hair growth.

Iron

Iron is another popular hair supplement. Very few cases of hair loss are directly related to iron deficiency, benefiting from taking iron supplements. Find out with your dermatologist if iron supplements are right for your hair loss. It will require baseline blood work showing either iron deficiency and/or low ferritin levels. After taking supplements for a few weeks or months, follow up with a blood test to determine the efficacy of the treatment in reversing the initial deficiency. Also, different forms of iron have varying absorption rates. I prefer ferronyl iron 65mg coupled with vitamin C 125mg to help with iron absorption. So, be sure to review all the above with your physician, establishing why you're taking iron supplements, for how long, how you will determine the success of your treatment and, most importantly, when you can stop. Don't take iron on a whim.

Vitamin D

Vitamin D deficiency can be associated with some forms of hair loss, specifically stubborn and severe forms of alopecia areata and some cases of telogen effluvium. Both forms of hair loss are usually reversible but require a specific approach. Having hair loss certainly *does not* equal having vitamin D deficiency or benefiting from vitamin D supplements. Blindly taking vitamin D can backfire as you may be over treating (rarely) or, what's far more common, undertreating your deficiency and not knowing when to stop or what to expect. Find out if you need to take vitamin D and determine what your end point is, i.e., when can you stop taking it.

Chapter 10: The Sun Guide

Let's address the elephant in the room. *Many* dermatologists, academics, as well as healthcare policymakers and influencers consider sunlight a human carcinogen first and then everything else. Studies back this, associating exposure to sunlight, and ultraviolet radiation (UVR) with DNA damage, cell damage, tissue damage, and increased incidence of skin cancer. This is not the whole story, and the validity of most studies are questionable on various grounds.

Despite controversy, the narrative strongly associating UVR with skin cancer in unquestionable and almost absolute terms presently dominates the institutions, including academia, healthcare, and government. This leads to statements such the one on the American Academy of Dermatology FAQs regarding everyone requiring sunblock or the FDA declaring: "There is no such thing as a **safe** tan.[79] The increase in skin pigment, called melanin, which causes the tan color change in your skin is a sign of damage."[80] This is an absolutist statement, rather than a measured and reasonable approach.

Consider this: In European populations, the incidence and mortality rates of malignant melanoma (MM) were 11.2 and 1.7 per 100,000/year, respectively, which is 0.0112 percent and 0.0017 percent of the population. In the U.S., those rates are 12.2 and 1.4 per 100,000/year (0.0122 percent and 0.0014 percent) and in Australia and New Zealand the rates are 33.6 and 3.4 (0.0336 percent and 0.0034 percent) per 100,000/year.[81] Mortality rates from squamous cell carcinoma (SCC) of the skin are estimated at around 0.52 per 100,000 in the U.S.[82] with rates three times higher in men than in women, as well as three times higher in whites compared with blacks. These are rough estimates but indicate the extent of the issue.

Sunlight, as well as UVR have important biological roles, not to be underestimated or ignored. Exposure to UVR contributing to carcinogenesis in some cases is the exception, not the rule. In fact, UVR can activate a category of mechanisms called autophagy leading to apoptosis, i.e., self-destruction of defective cells,[83] possibly contributing to cancer prevention. All human beings benefit from sunlight, directly through effects on the skin and the body, including vitamin D production, production of nitric oxide, improving mental health, as well as indirectly through effects on other people, animals, plants, and so on.

Long-term sun exposure also associates with protective effects for several types of cancer, including breast, colon, prostate, and non-Hodgkin's lymphoma[84] as well as chronic disease such as diabetes mellitus, hypertension, and multiple sclerosis.[85] The overwhelming majority of people on the planet do not get skin cancer, including people of European descent. The risk for developing sun damage and, more rarely, skin cancer are an individual matter. Now, while it is not the rule, excessive UVR exposure *can contribute* to carcinogenesis. The association is stronger in people who possess certain characteristics, such as fair skin; blue, green, or hazel eyes; red hair; and other factors. While skin cancer is common compared with other cancers, advanced cancer or skin cancer-related death is relatively uncommon. However, sunlight, including UVR is essential for people,[86] even those who have had skin cancer. They still need to produce vitamin D in their skin, as well as benefit from other effects of sunlight on their skin.

I think designating UVR (or sunlight) as a carcinogen is a mistake. I regard UVR and sunlight as essential natural phenomena of great biological significance (much of which is likely undiscovered), which may contribute to skin aging, and more rarely, to carcinogenesis.

I do not subscribe to the collectivist approach asserting everyone needs to use sunblock or "no such thing as a safe tan." This is nothing more than a moral panic masquerading as a rational and learned opinion. It is a generalizing assertion, which deprives the trusting public from realizing the nuance of sun exposure with regard to benefits and risks, as well as applicability to the individual considering one's personal traits, such as ability to tan.

This means determining the right balance of sun exposure is crucial, requiring some experimentation with one's own skin. For those who would like to avoid sunburn or even tanning at all costs, I've got some bad news and some good news.

The Bad News of Sun Trial and Error

The bad news is you and/or your child *may* experience sunburn and will almost certainly tan. You *can* avoid sunburn by incrementally and carefully increasing sun exposure. Older family members — parents or older siblings with similar skin tone — give some indication as for how the skin will react. They can provide some information regarding the time it takes to go from suntan to sunburn. Hopefully, you can completely avoid sunburn episodes or limit them to a handful of light burns. Tanning will likely happen repeatedly.

The Good News of Sun Trial and Error

The good news: With tanning or even burning, there are lessons about the limits of your skin's tolerance to sunlight and UVR, including determining how long it takes to tan, burn, and at what times of day. I am not advocating you purposefully set out to sunburn. Far from it. However, with a few exceptions, such as extreme sensitivity to sunlight such as genetic conditions, you must and should experiment with sun exposure.

Why? Because sunlight is essential for human health, and in excess can lead to sunburn, which is injurious to the skin. It is indispensable and when unchecked it can cause problems, so you must know what your sun limitations are. This is true for many other important aspects of life, and why you should have a close intimate knowledge of your relationship to the sun and its effects. You need to know how much is enough, and what's too much. The only way to know is to experiment. And because the sun is crucial, don't sit this one out.

So Now What?

What is the right degree of exposure? It's for you to figure it out for yourself. How does one figure out what's too much sun exposure? First, let's define what excessive sun exposure or sunburn looks like. Sunburn is injurious to the skin and associated with symptoms and sensations that are akin to irritation much like any other burn, such as redness, flakiness, blistering, itch, burning, and pain, giving you several indications.

I encourage establishing your sun exposure boundaries. Find your threshold for tanning using it as a ruler to judge the degree of sun exposure you can handle. So, your level of sun exposure should ideally amount to getting a light tan, and completely avoid sunburn on its various levels.

Dr. Michael F. Holick is a physician and a scientist who has been investigating the role of vitamin D, its benefits, and its relationship to sun exposure for over forty years. I spoke with Dr. Holick[87] to understand how sun exposure wound up as a demon on such a wide scale. According to Dr. Holick, the trend began with the association of sun exposure with skin cancer. Once the medical world made the connection, it became the center of the conversation in academia, among healthcare professionals, and further supported by the skincare industry, which stood to gain by selling sunblock. Despite increasing evidence of numerous benefits of sun exposure to human health, the "C" word trumped all other considerations. Skin cancer concerns, rather than a more holistic cost-benefit approach, continue to dictate institutional guidelines around the world.

In the course of his work, Dr. Holick has developed the nuanced concept he termed "sensible sun exposure." This is a refined approach Dr. Holick has formulated to empower individuals to define what degree of sun exposure they need to get the required vitamin D dose.

Per the sensible sun exposure prescription, estimate how long it takes for you to get a mild sunburn (known as one minimal erythemal dose, or 1MED), i.e., the appearance of a light pinkness over the exposed areas a day after sun exposure. Then, without applying sunscreen, expose your hands, arms, and face for 25 percent 1MED (or your arms and legs if you want to minimize facial wrinkling). According to Dr. Holick, the amount of sun exposure two to three days a week enables the body to make enough vitamin D to keep healthy. After spending the prescribed amount of time without protection, Dr. Holick recommends employing sun protection to prevent sun damage. Naturally, the more skin you expose to the sun, the more vitamin D you make. If you are wearing a swimsuit, it will take you less time per exposure than 25 percent of 1MED to make the minimum amount of vitamin D you need. It doesn't matter which area of your body gets the sun so long as at least 25 percent is.

Dr. Holick partnered with a California company called ontometrics, which produced an app, which could help determine when and how much sun exposure one needs based on your geographic location, body type, and time of day, while making sure you avoid injury by warning you of any risk sunburn. If you'd like to learn more, check out its website.[88]

Dr. Han van der Rhee is a Dutch dermatologist who started out as a staunch advocate of strict and aggressive sun protection. However, in the late 2000s, Dr. van der Rhee began to grow critical of the generalizing sun protective approach adopted by various institutions without much thought given to the advantages of sun exposure.[89] Similarly to my own experience as well as other dermatologists I've spoken to, Dr. van der Rhee recalls the beginning of his departure from convention by not adhering to institutional recommendations himself. His take on sun exposure is pragmatic and reminiscent of Dr. Holick's approach, focusing on personal skin qualities, one's relationship with sun exposure, and tendency to tan and burn. Much like Holick, Dr. van der Rhee describes professional and institutional backlash to his views, which appeared to stem from emotion and dogmatic thought rather than addressing his claims.

There are likely several reasons for the backlash met by the above dissidents who have done nothing more than challenge the conventional narrative or institutional orthodoxy. In my opinion, the main reason is deep convictions held by a critical and vocal mass of dermatologists and establishment bureaucrats framing ultraviolet light as a carcinogen, and exclusively feared rather than holistically respected. This belief coupled with the *perceived* role as a physician (or even a bureaucrat) with the fiduciary responsibility to one's patients creates the conditions for a fierce reaction when someone challenges the dogma. What's often overlooked is the responsibility to reexamine views and beliefs guiding the fiduciary. Actions not titles account for meeting fiduciary responsibilities.

With sunblock manufacturers, strong financial incentives likely play a significant role in SIC promotion of sun protection and the heavy-handed movement against sun exposure, couched as a healthcare campaign.

Sensible Sun Exposure — Sun Skinese

All methods of sun protection, especially sunblock, are inherently limited. There is no complete protection from UVR once exposed to sunlight, regardless of the type of sunblock you use. Sunblock is not a lead shield. This means when using any method of sun protection, one must determine how effective this method is and play within the parameters. Specifically, understand the timeframe in which a sun protection method expires or stops being effective at which point your skin will start tanning, and possibly even burn. Moreover, sunblock filters out some parts of the UV spectrum and allows in others. While the spectrum of UV filtration by sunblock has broadened, there remain many questions about the degree of differential efficacy of blockage, i.e., how much of each blocked wavelength gets through.

The best way to avoid sun damage is to time your exposure to get as much as you need, and then stop. If you stay in the sun past getting a tan and cannot physically protect yourself, I recommend using a topical sunblock. Obviously, the above scenario is not realistic. In life, we simply can neither completely stay away from the sun, time every exposure, nor always find shelter from the sun. You are better off having a healthy balanced approach to sun exposure, so it doesn't become a crippling obsession.

Sunblock

Topical sunblock is a versatile category of products, including sprays, lotions, creams, and more. Broadly, UVR blockers divide into organic chemical blockers and inorganic blockers, also known as physical blockers, which include zinc oxide, titanium dioxide. Many countries regulate sunscreen's active ingredients, including the United States by the FDA. Government bureaucrats consider research and available data on those chemicals and certify them either as "generally recognized as safe and effective" (GRASE) or not GRASE[90], with several inherent drawbacks. For example, the certification is only as good as the information available, the bureaucrats' comprehension of the data, as well as their good faith. Even if bureaucrats had prioritized "safety and efficacy" above all and had full comprehension of all available data, the breadth of data would still limit us, as well as the futility of generalizing what is safe and effective for every single person. Definition of safe and effective is a dynamic one and keeps shifting with data, as well as our growing understanding of skin.

Another obvious limitation to government bureaucracy is its pace and inefficiency. An individual can immediately stop using a product containing an ingredient deemed or suspected dangerous. The bureaucracy may take weeks, months, or even years to publish its own verdict. This is understandable since we expect the bureaucracy to deliberate decisions thoroughly, incorporating more knowledge and expertise than the average person. But bureaucracies have a way of wasting time and resources leading to a slow and stunned action, while the public image of a suspect ingredient may remain favorable due to this delay.

Effects on the microbiome of most sunblock ingredients are unknown. However, there are some reports of titanium dioxide and zinc oxide affecting the gut microbiome.[91] If you must use sunblock, apply a thin layer over exposed body parts and remember to reapply at least every two to three hours for continued effect. Some products incorporate iron oxide which is a visible sunlight blocker, which is applicable in people with melasma.

Personally, I don't use much sunblock and try to restrict use to face, ears, and the neck, using zinc oxide/titanium dioxide products, strictly when I expect to spend longer than ideal out in the open and have no other choice of covering appropriately or getting away from the sun. Obviously, nothing is ever perfect.

Skin Cancer Screening

I consider awareness and screening of skin cancer far more important than obsessing with sun avoidance. Skin cancer awareness increases agency, keeping you alert, focused, prompting you to act when you suspect something is up.

Campaigns over the past few decades aimed at raising public mindfulness to skin cancer, specifically MM. The ABCDEs of skin cancer help to discern the suspicious melanocytic lesion from the regular. The ABCDEs stand for the following:

A – Asymmetry – Benign lesions are frequently symmetrical, round, or oval. Many skin cancers, especially MM, or atypical moles are irregularly or bizarrely shaped.

B – Borders – Lesions have clear and distinct borders or edges. Some skin cancers have fuzzy or poorly defined borders, which could indicate the lesion is expanding.

C – Color – Many benign lesions are regularly colored, typically either uniformly — brown, tan, red, etc. — or the colors symmetrically distribute as concentric circles (bullseye pattern) for example.

D – Diameter – Skin cancer characteristics are by cell proliferation and growth, with many of them (not all) larger than other lesions on the skin. The diameter typically mentioned is anything beyond 6mm, an arbitrary cutoff that I think is most helpful when coupled with growth dynamics.

E – Evolution – This refers to active and ongoing growth or other changes in the appearance of the lesion, whether it's increasing in size, changes in the shape of a lesion, blurring borders, or changing colors.

I often tell my patients to urgently come in for evaluation with any suspicious lesion and don't care how banal it'll seem in hindsight. Whether one can explain why a lesion is suspicious is irrelevant, with some skin cancers appearing unremarkable, and some benign lesions appearing irregular.

The campaigns didn't address the nuance of skin cancer, which could mean the difference between life and death. Here are the most common misunderstandings I've encountered regarding skin cancer, all of which could lead to delaying or failing to seek medical attention.

Skin Cancer Can Be Flat or Raised

Skin cancers and some pre-cancerous lesions come in many forms, some flat, i.e., not rough, gritty, bumpy, or raised, meaning the lesion in question can appear as a blotch on the skin, with the same texture as the surrounding skin. Specifically, pre-cancerous lesions such as severely dysplastic nevi (moles), as well as skin cancers known as malignant melanoma in-situ, lentigo maligna melanoma, superficially spreading malignant melanoma, and acral lentiginous melanoma (ALM, which usually develops on palms or feet in areas *not* typically exposed to sun) can appear as flat irregularly shaped blemishes of varying sizes and colors. Colors range from different shades of brown, black, blue, red, pink, or even white, often unevenly distributed throughout the lesion.

Skin Cancers Can Appear on Any Part of the Skin

Flat lesions go unnoticed, especially when appearing on body parts not commonly self-examined, e.g., scalp, mouth, privates, backside, palms, soles, and toenails. Moreover, *any* type of skin cancer can appear anywhere on the body, requiring examining those areas periodically.

Some Skin Cancers Are Not Sun Related

Another consequence of the awareness campaigns is focusing on skin cancers on sun-exposed areas. However, in many cases pre-cancerous lesions and skin cancers can develop over areas that are not typically sun exposed. This is more common among people of African, Southeast Asian, and South American descent. As previously mentioned, the musician Bob Marley died of a metastatic ALM, which originated on his toe. So, not all skin cancers are created equal, requiring examining literally the *entire* body when looking for them.

Some Skin Cancers Appear as Chronic Ulcers

Chronic ulcers or sores are a very common problem, often developing after trauma to a vulnerable area, such as legs or feet, but affecting practically any area of the body. Skin cancers, including squamous cell carcinomas (SCC), basal cell carcinomas (BCC) and MM can appear as ulcers, even in early stages. Moreover, skin cancer represents abnormal tissue, meaning in many cases it is more fragile than normal skin, and more prone to ulcerating. While *most* sores or ulcers are *not* cancer, some are.

If you have a sore or a crusty area unusually persisting for more than a couple of weeks, consult a board-certified dermatologist. Even if it is not skin cancer, the dermatologist must follow chronic ulcers and often treat intentionally and aggressively. A non-healing ulcer can spell big trouble, especially on the legs and feet, and even more so with immune compromising conditions such as diabetes mellitus.

Some People Explain Away Their Skin Cancers

Numerous times I've diagnosed skin cancers in lesions patients thought were nothing, i.e., nothing to worry about. Most frequently the cancerous lesion is flat and develops on a hard to see area, such as the back. However, the cancer is often either on the face, arm, or leg, in plain sight, yet the patient seems oblivious to it. Usually, it is not straight denial, but rather a story explaining how the lesion appeared. The stories make sense on some level and may have a grain of truth. Here are a few examples.

Skin cancer stories from the frontlines of the Greater Boston Metro area:

Joe, *a 73-year-old retired Boston Police Department officer, his once-upon-a-time fair skin marred by long decades of sun damage, came by to see me for a skin exam at my Fenway Park office. As I was examining his skin, I spotted a 1cm ulcer on the right forearm that turned out to be an SCC. When I asked Joe about the ulcer, he seemed to minimize the finding. His explanation: "Oh, this sore? I banged into a door a few weeks ago. It almost disappeared and then I picked at it, so it opened back up again."*

Bridgette, *a 53-year-old executive assistant and a Cambridge resident, came by to "burn" a few annoying spots on her face, when I noticed a 3mm ulcerated "pimple" on the nasal bridge that turned out to be a BCC. Bridgette's explanation: "I got a new pair of reading glasses a couple of months ago, and they irritated my nose. Also, I think I may have scratched it, so it keeps bleeding."*

Jean, *a 65-year-old retiree from Dorchester came by for a first-time skin exam at my Boston Medical Center clinic. Nothing to write home about, except for a large Band-Aid on her left ankle, which she assured me was nothing. When I inquired further, Jean explained: "I'm breaking in this new pair of leather shoes I bought about four months ago. They chafed my ankle." I asked Jean to take a look for myself, which she accepted. I removed the Band-Aid to reveal a 4cm ulcer, which turned out to be an MM.*

Owen, *a 65-year-old lawyer from Boston's South End, came by for treatment of warts on his hands. He declined a full skin exam but was OK with looking at his sun exposed areas, which led me to find a 5mm bump on the cheek, which turned out to be a BCC. Owen's explanation: "This pimple? I've had this for a few months. I couldn't help trying to pop it, so I think I made it mad."*

Now, the patients may be completely in the right regarding the history. As I mentioned before, skin cancer forms abnormal skin that can be very fragile and more prone to ulceration when traumatized or even form a sore spontaneously. Also, squeezing a pimple can prolong its healing. Those stories make sense in the right context. However, there is a difference between what sounds plausible and the actual bottom-line. If you have a new sore, an irregular blemish, a "pimple," or any other unusual skin lesion persisting more than two to three weeks, I highly recommend an evaluation by a board-certified dermatologist. It can save your life or the life of a loved one, lead to more conservative treatment with early detection, or at least peace of mind.

Chapter 11: Miscellaneous

Herpes Simplex Viral Infection — The Essential Guide

- HSV infection is mostly a self-limiting, transient condition recurring over the same anatomical location.
- HSV *often* starts with a tingle or sting over the outbreak location, followed by grouped reddish bumps, turning into clear or yellowish blisters, forming sores, finally resolving with little to no scarring.
- Episodes usually last days to a few weeks. Chronic cases are suspicious for an underlying immune deficiency.
- The first episode can be very dramatic with fever, severe pain, lymphadenopathy, and extensive blistering, though most primary infections go unnoticed.
- A febrile illness, sunburn, surgical procedures, and other life stresses can trigger many outbreaks (hence the term cold sore).
- Topical treatments are almost completely useless but may help as moisturizers, meaning you're better off using a plain moisturizer.
- Oral antiviral therapy is useful to prevent or curb the severity of an impending episode.
- Suppressive oral therapy taken daily is useful in decreasing the number of outbreaks in people experiencing more than a handful of episodes a year.
- HSV infection is usually inconsequential becoming a problem in a handful of special circumstances: herpes keratitis, an infection of the eye that could lead to permanent damage; vertical transmission from mother to newborn, possibly leading to severe infection, permanent damage, and death; HSV in immunocompromised patients.

Not All Sores Are Cold Sores

Sores around or inside the mouth or genitals are often mistakenly lumped as cold sores or genital sores (meaning infectious), respectively. While HSV infection is common, there are many other possible causes for mouth or genital sores, requiring specific treatments. To clarify, sores not caused by HSV will not respond to antiviral treatments. Management *must* match the condition. Here are a few conditions leading to mouth ulcers.

- Canker sores or aphthous ulcers are painful lesions inside the mouth or privates, usually self-limiting. They are usually idiopathic but can be associated with other conditions. Prolonged cases require treatment and, sometimes, additional workup.
- HSV infection classically begins as grouped reddish bumps, which then turn into blisters, finally forming sores. It is mostly a self-limiting, transient condition, which recurs over the same anatomical location.
- Lichen planus (LP) is a chronic condition sometimes forming painful ulcers inside the mouth, genitals, as well as other parts of the skin.
- Pemphigus/pemphigoid is a category of autoimmune conditions causing skin and mucosal surfaces to blister, forming sores, many of which are painful, requiring medical attention and management.
- Oral or genital cancer, including squamous cell carcinoma, can be deadly, making early detection crucial.

Bottom line: If you're suffering from persistent or frequently occurring oral or genital ulcers, clarify your diagnosis and obtain the correct treatment for optimal results. See your board-certified dermatologist for management.

A Special Note on Face Masks

The COVID 19 scare-related widespread wearing of face masks, led to a pandemic of facial skin ailments, including itch, irritation, pimples, pustules, and more. While I can't replace a careful evaluation and management by your dermatologist, here are a few tips to keep in mind:

- Limit your face mask wearing to the absolute necessary minimum, avoiding it whenever possible.
- If you must use a mask, wear disposable face masks, ideally replacing them at least once a day, or whenever they become soaked with sweat, makeup, etc.
- If you must use cloth masks, wash them with lukewarm water *only* without detergent. Detergent soaked into masks can irritate your skin and adversely affect your microbiome.
- If you must use a detergent to wash your mask, consider using a laundry detergent free of fragrance and dyes.
- Avoid using antibiotic/antibacterial soaked masks.
- Choose masks made with smooth, soft, porous materials.
- If you must wash your face, do so solely with lukewarm water and be sure to moisturize as needed.
- Know your limitations. When dealing with persistent or worsening itching, burning, redness, flakiness, bumps, or whiteheads, limit conservative measures as above to seven to ten days. The spectrum of mask-related ailments is simply too versatile for a shotgun approach and wrong treatment can lead to a worsening in your condition.
- If your condition persists more than a week despite conservative measures, seek the advice of a board-certified dermatologist to evaluate and manage it accordingly.

Closing Thoughts

Congratulations! You've come a long way, from my own personal journey from a clueless wonder to a dermatologist, from inside the belly of the SIC beast, and finally to fundamentals, empowering you to understand your own skin. With the ending of this book, your own journey of a lifelong healthy relationship with your skin begins. It is not an easy journey, requiring perseverance and strength of character to stick with some of the recommendations made in this book, especially when just starting. Don't lose sight of the messages of the SIC around you, in your own habits, other people's habits, electronic media, social media, and traditional media. The SIC is in the air we breathe and the water we drink. The good news is once you know what to look for, you start seeing previously trusted assertions for what they are: utter and complete nonsense. Stay strong. Keep the faith. Practice your Skinese. And if you ever hit a snag, call me.

With immense gratitude,

Yuval Bibi, MD, PhD, Dermatologist

https://drbibiorganics.com

Additional Resources

For further information, special offers, updates, courses, and upcoming events stay connected at DrBibiOrganics.com

For offerings from Dr. Bibi including his book catalog, skincare products as well as a curated list of additional products and accessories meeting his exceptional commitment to minimalist skincare.
Drbibiorganics.com/pages/skincare

For the world's leading moisturizer personally engineered by Dr. Bibi.
Drbibiorganics.com/products/butter-oasis-moisturizing-balm

For ongoing video content on skincare, dermatology, medicine, healthcare, philosophy, religion and more go to youtube.com/@TheRogueDermatologist

For Dr. Bibi's groundbreaking book - *Baby Skincare: Skincare for Infants & Early Childhood* go to https://a.co/d/00tynzHj

About the Author

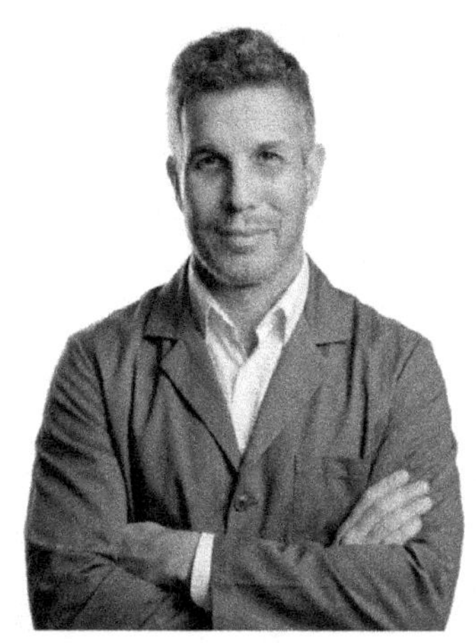

Dr. Yuval Bibi, MD, PhD, is a board-certified dermatologist with a PhD in neuroscience and postdoctoral training in cancer biology and innate immunology. In addition to bread-and-butter dermatology, he specializes in what many won't touch: scalp pathology, genital and oral skin disease, nail disorders—the conditions that require both nerve and precision. After clinical training at Boston University and Tufts, Dr. Bibi did something most physicians would consider insane: he moved to Los Angeles to pursue acting and screenwriting. Not as a hobby. As a career. He lived the volatility, wrote the scripts, learned what it means to rebuild your value from zero every single day.

During that period, he founded Dr. Bibi Organics, a vegan skincare line built on radical minimalism—strip away everything that doesn't serve you. In products. In medicine. In life.

This book was born from that rare vantage point: standing with one foot in clinical dermatology, the other in the skincare industry's glittering machinery. Dr. Bibi has seen what both worlds don't want you to know—how diagnoses get marketed as insecurities, how science gets bent into sales copy, how the space between health and commerce is where truth goes to die. He's writing from the fault line, and he's not interested in protecting either side.

Now practicing in South Florida, Dr. Bibi continues to operate at the intersection of science, storytelling, and helping his patients navigate the controlled chaos of skin and the human body with their eyes open and their heads held up high.

Dr. Bibi's approach is for those who refuse to be sold what they don't need, who demand answers instead of marketing, and who are ready to reclaim their skin—and their autonomy—from an industry built on fear and profit. This book is that reclamation.

.

End Notes

---

[1] From what I've seen, very few people do. I will address conditioning in detail in the hair guide in Chapter 9.

[2] https://www.nih.gov/news-events/news-releases/nih-human-microbiome-project-defines-normal-bacterial-makeup-body

[3] Rossen NG, MacDonald JK, de Vries EM, D'Haens GR, de Vos WM, Zoetendal EG, Ponsioen CY. Fecal microbiota transplantation as novel therapy in gastroenterology: A systematic review. World J Gastroenterol. 2015 May 7;21(17):5359-71. doi: 10.3748/wjg.v21.i17.5359. PMID: 25954111. PMCID: PMC4419078

[4] Adams JB, Borody TJ, Kang DW, Khoruts A, Krajmalnik-Brown R, Sadowsky MJ. Microbiota transplant therapy and autism: lessons for the clinic. Expert Rev Gastroenterol Hepatol. 2019 Nov;13(11):1033-1037. doi: 10.1080/17474124.2019.1687293. Epub 2019 Nov 7. PMID: 31665947

[5] Any inanimate object that, when contaminated with or exposed to infectious agents, can transfer disease to a new host.

[6] Castillo CR, Alishahedani ME, Gough P, Chaudhary PP, Yadav M, Matriz J, Myles IA. Assessing the effects of common topical exposures on skin bacteria associated with atopic dermatitis. Skin Health Dis. 2021 Sep;1(3):e41. doi: 10.1002/ski2.41. Epub 2021 May 7. PMID: 34723253; PMCID: PMC8555759

[7] Myles IA, Earland NJ, Anderson ED, Moore IN, Kieh MD, Williams KW, Saleem A, Fontecilla NM, Welch PA, Darnell DA, Barnhart LA, Sun AA, Uzel G, Datta SK. First-in-human topical microbiome transplantation with Roseomonas mucosa for atopic dermatitis. JCI Insight. 2018 May 3;3(9):e120608. doi: 10.1172/jci.insight.120608. PMID: 29720571; PMCID: PMC6012572

[8] AD, a condition characterized by sensitive skin and eczema

[9] Wang Q, Cui S, Zhou L, He K, Song L, Liang H, He C. Effect of cosmetic chemical preservatives on resident flora isolated from healthy facial skin. J Cosmet Dermatol. 2019 Apr;18(2):652-658. doi: 10.1111/jocd.12822. Epub 2018 Dec 12. PMID: 30548758

---

[10] Statista, https://www.statista.com/statistics/254612/global-skin-care-market-size/

[11] https://www.groupon.com/merchant/trends-insights/market-research/true-cost-beauty-americans-spend-most-survey

[12] https://www.today.com/health/stop-obsessing-women-waste-2-weeks-year-their-appearance-today-2D12104866

[13] Known as apoptosis

[14] Eckhart L, Lippens S, Tschachler E, Declercq W. Cell death by cornification. Biochim Biophys Acta. 2013 Dec;1833(12):3471-3480. doi: 10.1016/j.bbamcr.2013.06.010. Epub 2013 Jun 20. PMID: 23792051

[15] Grice EA, Segre JA. The skin microbiome. Nat Rev Microbiol. 2011 Apr;9(4):244-53. doi: 10.1038/nrmicro2537. Erratum in: Nat Rev Microbiol. 2011 Aug;9(8):626. PMID: 21407241; PMCID: PMC3535073

[16] Burton M, Cobb E, Donachie P, Judah G, Curtis V, Schmidt WP. The effect of handwashing with water or soap on bacterial contamination of hands. Int J Environ Res Public Health. 2011 Jan;8(1):97-104. doi: 10.3390/ijerph8010097. Epub 2011 Jan 6. PMID: 21318017; PMCID: PMC3037063

[17] Voegeli D. The effect of washing and drying practices on skin barrier function. J Wound Ostomy Continence Nurs. 2008 Jan-Feb;35(1):84-90. doi: 10.1097/01.WON.0000308623.68582.d7. PMID: 18199943

[18] https://www.gallinee.com/our-story/

[19] https://www.wordnik.com/words/disinfection

[20] Relating to, applied to, or affecting a localized area of the body, especially of the skin. https://www.wordnik.com/words/topical

[21] Macpherson H, Pipingas A, Pase MP. Multivitamin-multimineral supplementation and mortality: a meta-analysis of randomized controlled trials. Am J Clin Nutr. 2013 Feb;97(2):437-44. doi: 10.3945/ajcn.112.049304. Epub 2012 Dec 19. PMID: 23255568

[22] Sekhri K, Kaur K. Public knowledge, use, and attitude toward multivitamin supplementation: A cross-sectional study among general public. Int J Appl Basic Med Res. 2014 Jul;4(2):77-80. doi: 10.4103/2229-516X.136780. PMID: 25143880; PMCID: PMC4137646

[23] Which are valuable despite the abuse.

[24] Cutaneous cleansers. Kuehl BL, Fyfe KS, Shear NH. Skin Therapy Lett. 2003 Mar;8(3):1-4.

[25] Otherwise known as xerosis

[26] An immensely complicated concept by itself

[27] A highly subjective term

[28] The observable physical or biochemical characteristics of an organism, as determined by both genetic makeup and environmental influences https://www.thefreedictionary.com/phenotypic

[29] https://www.aad.org/dw/dw-insights-and-inquiries/2019-archive/september/parabens

[30] Vindenes HK, Lin H, Shigdel R, Ringel-Kulka T, Real FG, Svanes C, Peddada SD, Bertelsen RJ. Exposure to Antibacterial Chemicals Is Associated with Altered Composition of Oral Microbiome. Front Microbiol. 2022 Apr 28;13:790496. doi: 10.3389/fmicb.2022.790496. PMID: 35572708; PMCID: PMC9096491

[31] Čepelak I, Dodig S, Pavić I. Filaggrin and atopic march. Biochem Med (Zagreb). 2019 Jun 15;29(2):020501. doi: 10.11613/BM.2019.020501. PMID: 31223255; PMCID: PMC6559618

[32] Weatherly LM, Shim J, Hashmi HN, Kennedy RH, Hess ST, Gosse JA. Antimicrobial agent triclosan is a proton ionophore uncoupler of mitochondria in living rat and human mast cells and in primary human keratinocytes. J Appl Toxicol. 2016 Jun;36(6):777-89. doi: 10.1002/jat.3209. Epub 2015 Jul 23. PMID: 26204821; PMCID: PMC4724348

[33] Dubey D, Chopra D, Singh J, Srivastav AK, Kumari S, Verma A, Ray RS. Photosensitized methyl paraben induces apoptosis via caspase dependent pathway under ambient UVB exposure in human skin cells. Food Chem Toxicol. 2017 Oct;108(Pt A):171-185. doi: 10.1016/j.fct.2017.07.056. Epub 2017 Jul 29. Erratum in: Food Chem Toxicol. 2018 Oct;120:729-730. PMID: 28764904

[34] Datta S, Baudouin C, Brignole-Baudouin F, Denoyer A, Cortopassi GA. The eye drop preservative benzalkonium chloride potently induces mitochondrial dysfunction and preferentially affects LHON mutant cells. Invest Ophthalmol Vis Sci.

2017 Apr 1;58(4):2406-2412. doi: 10.1167/iovs.16-20903. PMID: 28444329; PMCID: PMC5407244

[35] https://ph.pg.com/product-safety/

[36] https://olay.co.uk/skin-care-products/face-moisturiser/regenerist-3-point-firming-treatment-cream

[37] https://www.olay.com/en-us/skin-care-products/regenerist-micro-sculpting-cream-moisturizer

[38] This claim is in regard to multiple Regenerist products

[39] We're not told which peptides P&G is using but here is a possible candidate: Palmitoyl Pentapeptide-4 (truthinaging.com)

[40] https://www.cosmeticsinfo.org/whats-in-my-products/ingredient-alphabetical/

[41] https://cosmetics.specialchem.com/selectors

[42] D. Gordon Smith, The Critical Resource Theory of Fiduciary Duty, 55 VAND. L. REV. 1399 (2002)

[43] https://www.aquaphorus.com/products/body-care/healing-ointment

[44] https://www.olay.com/en-us/skin-care-products/olay-regenerist-whip-face-moisturizer-spf-25

[45] https://www.cerave.com/skincare/moisturizers/healing-ointment

[46] https://en.wikipedia.org/wiki/Science

[47] Baker M. 1,500 scientists lift the lid on reproducibility. Nature. 2016 May 26;533(7604):452-4. doi: 10.1038/533452a. PMID: 27225100

[48] The Pepsodent Effect — the experience-based skincare promotion leading to habit formation

[49] Canavez ADPM, de Oliveira Prado Corrêa G, Isaac VLB, Schuck DC, Lorencini M. Integrated approaches to testing and assessment as a tool for the hazard assessment and risk characterization of cosmetic preservatives. J Appl Toxicol. 2021 Oct;41(10):1687-1699. doi: 10.1002/jat.4156. Epub 2021 Feb 24. PMID: 33624850.

---

[50] https://www.fda.gov/cosmetics/cosmetics-science-research/product-testing-cosmetics

[51] For example, see P&G website.

[52] Vivek Ramaswami, Woke Inc. 2021, Center Street/Hachette Book Group.

[53] https://www.ncbi.nlm.nih.gov/pmc/articles/PMC7859136/#CR15; https://pubmed.ncbi.nlm.nih.gov/34343557/

[54] Hill, SE, Christopher D, Griskevicius, Vladas, Durante, K, White, AE. Boosting beauty in an economic decline: mating, spending, and the lipstick effect J Pers Soc Psychol. 2012 Aug;103(2):275-91. doi: 10.1037/a0028657. Epub 2012 May 28

[55] tonyrobbins.com

[56] https://hookagency.com/blog/pepsodent-ad-habit/

[57] Levy SB. Antibacterial household products: cause for concern. emerging infectious diseases. 2001;7(7):512-515. doi:10.3201/eid0707.017705. See: https://wwwnc.cdc.gov/eid/article/7/7/01-7705_article

[58] https://www.fda.gov/news-events/press-announcements/fda-issues-final-rule-safety-and-effectiveness-antibacterial-soaps

[59] Vandegrift R, Bateman AC, Siemens KN, Nguyen M, Wilson HE, Green JL, Van Den Wymelenberg KG, Hickey RJ. Cleanliness in context: reconciling hygiene with a modern microbial perspective. Microbiome. 2017 Jul 14;5(1):76. doi: 10.1186/s40168-017-0294-2. PMID: 28705228; PMCID: PMC5513348

[60] For example: Aiello AE, Larson EL, Levy SB. Consumer antibacterial soaps: effective or just risky? Clin Infect Dis. 2007 Sep 1;45 Suppl 2:S137-47. doi: 10.1086/519255. PMID: 1768301

[61] Meadow JF, Altrichter AE, Bateman AC, Stenson J, Brown GZ, Green JL, Bohannan BJ. Humans differ in their personal microbial cloud. PeerJ. 2015 Sep 22;3:e1258. doi: 10.7717/peerj.1258. PMID: 26417541; PMCID: PMC4582947

[62] Rocha LA, Ferreira de Almeida E Borges L, Gontijo Filho PP. Changes in hands microbiota associated with skin damage because of hand hygiene procedures on the health care workers. Am J Infect Control. 2009 Mar;37(2):155-9. doi: 10.1016/j.ajic.2008.04.251. PMID: 19249642

[63] Yu JJ, Manus MB, Mueller O, Windsor SC, Horvath JE, Nunn CL. Antibacterial soap use impacts skin microbial communities in rural Madagascar. PLoS One. 2018 Aug 20;13(8):e0199899. doi: 10.1371/journal.pone.0199899. PMID: 30125279; PMCID: PMC6101359

[64] Mukherjee PK, Chandra J, Retuerto M, Arters KA, Consolo MC, Patterson A, Bajaksouzian S, Arbogast JW, Cartner TJ, Jacobs MR, Ghannoum MA, Salata RA. Effect of alcohol-based hand rub on hand microbiome and hand skin health in hospitalized adult stem cell transplant patients: A pilot study. J Am Acad Dermatol. 2018 Jun;78(6):1218-1221.e5. doi: 10.1016/j.jaad.2017.11.046. Epub 2017 Dec 1. PMID: 29203437; PMCID: PMC5951739

[65] Zapka C, Leff J, Henley J, Tittl J, De Nardo E, Butler M, Griggs R, Fierer N, Edmonds-Wilson S. Comparison of standard culture-based method to culture-independent method for evaluation of hygiene effects on the hand microbiome. mBio. 2017 Mar 28;8(2):e00093-17. doi: 10.1128/mBio.00093-17. PMID: 28351915; PMCID: PMC5371408

[66] Strachan DP. Hay fever, hygiene, and household size. BMJ. 1989 Nov 18;299(6710):1259-60. doi: 10.1136/bmj.299.6710.1259. PMID: 2513902; PMCID: PMC1838109

[67] Professional associations, skincare professionals, influencers, etc.

[68] https://www.sciencedirect.com/science/article/pii/S0025326X20310018

[69] https://www.fda.gov/cosmetics/cosmetics-laws-regulations/microbead-free-waters-act-faqs

[70] https://www.plasticsoupfoundation.org/en/2021/01/cosmetics-industry-misleads-consumers-and-government-microbeads-in-personal-care-products-are-not-phased-out-at-all/

[71] South China Morning Post: https://www.scmp.com/news/people-culture/gender-diversity/article/3171868/if-you-dont-believe-it-smell-it-pg-apologises?module=perpetual_scroll_0&pgtype=article&campaign=3171868

[72] Charlie Specht. Mar 6, 2022, Updated May 4, 2022. https://buffalonews.com/news/local/nearly-500-women-owned-businesses-rejected-from-mwbe-program-but-ny-denies-fraud-concerns/article_7529f59e-997c-11ec-abea-fbac9cc284bc.html, *The Buffalo News*

---

[73] Steven Koprince. March 8, 2013. false wosb self-certifications potentially rampant, says NASA OIG. https://smallgovcon.com/debarment-and-penalties/false-wosb-self-certifications-potentially-rampant-says-nasa-oig/, *SmallGovCon*

[74] Yes, I know this is a loaded term. Ideally, a product with as few ingredients as possible and little to no reported side effects

[75] arising spontaneously or from an obscure or unknown cause, https://www.merriam-webster.com/dictionary/idiopathic

[76] Alopecia is a blanket term for hair loss

[77] Lubov, J. E., Okereke, U. R., Clapp, B., Toyohara, J., Taiwò, D., Kakpovbia, E., Lo Sicco, K., & Adotama, P. (2023). Central centrifugal cicatricial alopecia in Black men: A case series highlighting key clinical features in this cohort. JAAD Case Rep, 38, 27-31. doi: 10.1016/j.jdcr.2023.05.026.

[78] Perez-Sanchez AC, Burns EK, Perez VM, Tantry EK, Prabhu S, Katta R. Safety concerns of skin, hair and nail supplements in retail stores. Cureus. 2020 Jul 30;12(7):e9477. doi: 10.7759/cureus.9477. PMID: 32874806; PMCID: PMC7455464.

[79] Underlined and bolded by author

[80] https://www.fda.gov/radiation-emitting-products/tanning/risks-tanning

[81] Raimondi S, Suppa M, Gandini S. Melanoma epidemiology and sun exposure. Acta Derm Venereol. 2020 Jun 3;100(11):adv00136. doi: 10.2340/00015555-3491. PMID: 32346751

[82] Green AC, Olsen CM. Cutaneous squamous cell carcinoma: an epidemiological review. Br J Dermatol. 2017 Aug;177(2):373-381. doi: 10.1111/bjd.15324. Epub 2017 Feb 16. PMID: 28211039

[83] Sample A, He YY. Autophagy in UV Damage Response. Photochem Photobiol. 2017 Jul;93(4):943-955. doi: 10.1111/php.12691. Epub 2017 Jan 27. PMID: 27935061; PMCID: PMC5466513.

[84] van der Rhee H, Coebergh JW, de Vries E. Is prevention of cancer by sun exposure more than just the effect of vitamin D? A systematic review of epidemiological studies. Eur J Cancer. 2013 Apr;49(6):1422-36. doi: 10.1016/j.ejca.2012.11.001. Epub 2012 Dec 10. PMID: 23237739

---

[85] van der Rhee HJ, de Vries E, Coebergh JW. Regular sun exposure benefits health. Med Hypotheses. 2016 Dec;97:34-37. doi: 10.1016/j.mehy.2016.10.011. Epub 2016 Oct 19. PMID: 27876126

[86] There are exceptionally rare genetic conditions such as xeroderma pigmentosum and porphyria with which great caution and professional guidance is advised

[87] Personal interview conducted with Dr. Michael Holick by phone

[88] https://dminder.ontometrics.com/index.html. I have no business or personal relationship with ontometrics. This is not an endorsement or recommendation to purchase or use their product. I encourage you to do your due diligence

[89] Personal interview conducted with Dr. van der Rhee by phone

[90] https://www.fda.gov/drugs/news-events-human-drugs/update-sunscreen-requirements-deemed-final-order-and-proposed-order

[91] Ghebretatios M, Schaly S, Prakash S. Nanoparticles in the food industry and their impact on human gut microbiome and diseases. Int J Mol Sci. 2021 Feb 16;22(4):1942. doi: 10.3390/ijms22041942. PMID: 33669290; PMCID: PMC7920074

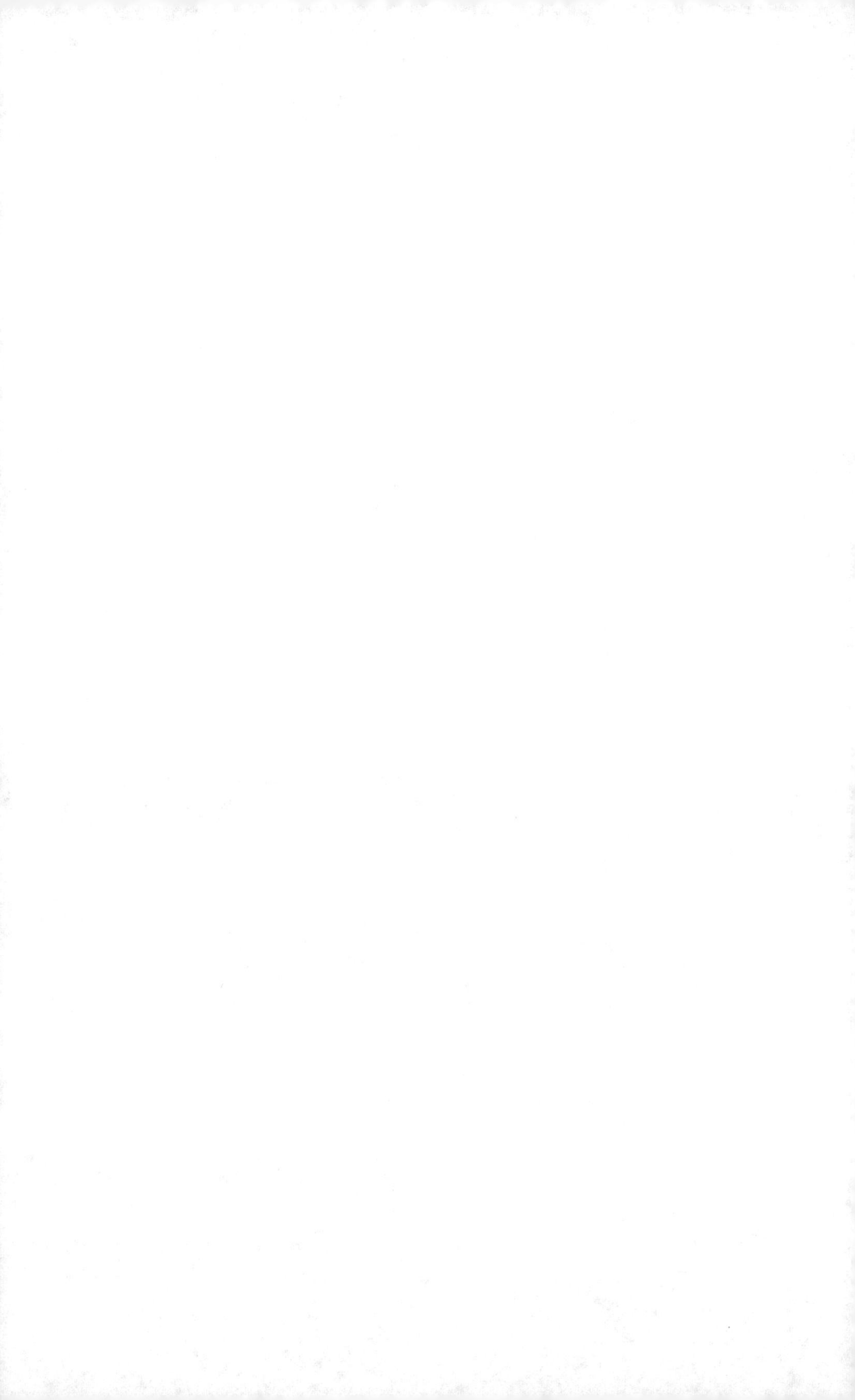

www.ingramcontent.com/pod-product-compliance
Lightning Source LLC
LaVergne TN
LVHW010915110826
845149LV00013B/2366

* 9 7 8 1 9 9 0 8 3 0 2 9 7 *